T0292553

# Digital Breast Tomosynthesis

Alberto Tagliafico
Nehmat Houssami • Massimo Calabrese
Editors

# Digital Breast Tomosynthesis

## A Practical Approach

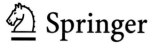 Springer

*Editors*
Alberto Tagliafico
Department of Experimental Medicine
University of Genova
Genova
Italy

Massimo Calabrese
Department of Diagnostic Senology
San Martino Hospital
Genova
Italy

Nehmat Houssami
School of Public Health
University of Sydney
Sydney
Australia

Electronic supplementary material is available in the online version of chapter 5 on SpringerLink: http://link.springer.com/

ISBN 978-3-319-28629-7      ISBN 978-3-319-28631-0   (eBook)
DOI 10.1007/978-3-319-28631-0

Library of Congress Control Number: 2016935928

Printed on acid-free paper

This Springer imprint is published by Springer Nature
The registered company is Springer International Publishing AG Switzerland

# Preface

Digital breast tomosynthesis (DBT) is emerging as an important imaging modality for both the screening and diagnosis of breast cancer. DBT improves on the capability of mammography by depicting breast tissue in three dimensions, hence overcoming the limitation of standard mammography, which can display only two-dimensional images. Yet, because it is essentially a re-invention of mammography, there is a familiarity in many aspects of DBT from a reader's perspective that makes it both appealing and feasible to learn and use in breast imaging practice. In clinical practice, DBT is read as video clips of cross-sectional images, reconstructed according to their mammographic planes of acquisition. Hence, in this book we present more than 30 video clips of DBT taken from our daily clinical practice to contribute practical knowledge to this emerging field. The goal is to introduce the beginner to DBT and to help physicians with more extensive experience in using DBT to consolidate their expertise.

This book aims to provide a description of screening and clinical applications of DBT and to offer simple and clear guidance on the technique. In the first chapter, Gisella Gennaro presents a brief overview of the physical principles of DBT. In the following chapters, Per Skaane assesses the potential of DBT in screening practice and Luca Carbonaro describes the clinical applications of DBT for various clinical indications. The final chapter includes clinical cases for didactic and practical learning, which is the focus of this book. These cases are taken from our daily clinical practice, where we perform 15 000 mammographic examinations, 10 000 DBTs, 5000 ultrasound scans, 500 magnetic resonance examinations, and 2300 biopsies per year. There is also a brief chapter discussing breast density overall and in relation to DBT.

We expect that by time this book is published, scientific publications and clinical evidence on the use of DBT will have increased rapidly. Therefore, we believe that this book is timely and provides a practical approach to enhancing knowledge on the use of DBT in clinical practice. We would like to thank all contributing authors for their time and contributions and for sharing their expertise in this volume. Contributing authors have a strong commitment to clinical and translational research in DBT, and are active researchers and teachers. We consider this aspect very important in creating a well-balanced, up-to-date, and useful text. Lead authors of the individual chapters were invited to share their insights because of their outstanding experience and major contributions to the radiological literature on the topic.

Finally, we would also like to thank in advance our readers and colleagues for whom we decided to develop this work.

Genova, Italy                                                              Alberto Tagliafico
Sydney, Australia                                                       Nehmat Houssami
Genova, Italy                                                          Massimo Calabrese

# Contents

# Physics and Radiation Dose of Digital Breast Tomosynthesis

**1**

Gisella Gennaro

## 1.1 Physical Principle of Tomosynthesis

Digital breast tomosynthesis (DBT) was proved to be feasible at the end of the 1990s, when digital mammography systems were going to be launched into the market (Niklason et al. 1997). It was already known that 2D mammography, despite the advent of new detectors, is inherently limited because of the superimposition of both normal and pathological structures when a transmission X-ray image is acquired. In fact, in mammography the 3D breast structure is projected onto the detector plane perpendicular to the X-ray source, and the multiple tissues and structures appear overlapped in the projection image. This has two effects on radiologists' capability of detecting subtle lesions in mammography images: on one side, malignant lesions might be masked by the presence of overlapped glandular tissue, producing false negatives; on the other side, the superimposition of normal tissues might determine false positives. The lowering of sensitivity and specificity in conventional mammography caused by tissue superimposition is often called "anatomical" or "structure" noise, i.e., something which is an obstacle for radiologists to correctly interpret image contents (Niklason et al. 1997; Burgess et al. 2001). The adverse effects of the anatomical noise can be reduced by introducing tomographic imaging methods, like tomosynthesis.

DBT is a quasi-3D imaging technique, which reconstructs tomographic images of the breast from a series of low-dose projection images acquired by a digital detector while the X-ray tube rotates within a limited arc (Park et al. 2007). This can be relatively easily obtained from a standard digital mammography platform where the gantry is allowed to move around an axis located above the breast support, while the digital detector remains stationary during the acquisition of the low-dose projection. Breast positioning in tomosynthesis is the same as used for conventional digital

G. Gennaro
Department of Radiology, Veneto Institute of Oncology (IOV) – IRCCS, Padova, Italy
e-mail: gisella.gennaro@ioveneto.it

© Springer International Publishing Switzerland 2016
A. Tagliafico et al. (eds.), *Digital Breast Tomosynthesis: A Practical Approach*,
DOI 10.1007/978-3-319-28631-0_1

mammography, with the breast compressed on the breast support to obtain different views (typically cranio-caudal, CC and mediolateral oblique, MLO) (Yaffe et al. 2014).

A schematic view of acquisition and reconstruction in digital breast tomosynthesis is depicted in Fig. 1.1a, b (Reiser et al. 2014).

The two objects (red and blue) within the breast are located along the $z$-axis at different depths, A and B. In DBT multiple projection images at low dose are acquired, with the X-ray source at different angles. The two objects appear overlapped in the central projection, but they are separated in the angled projections, with a shift proportional to the tube angle (Fig. 1.1a). The acquisition scheme is simplified for three projections, but in real DBT systems, the number of projection ranges between 9 and 25, depending on the system. In Fig. 1.1b the reconstruction process is illustrated, showing the result of a shift-and-add (SAA) algorithm. Multiple planes corresponding to different depths in the breast are reconstructed by adding the contribution of all the acquired low-dose projection images. For each reconstructed plane, the algorithm permits to have in focus only the structures belonging to that plane, while any other structure located in different planes is blurred. The reconstruction process, blurring everything comes from an out-of-focus plane, reduces the anatomical noise and favorites easier lesion detection (Reiser et al. 2014).

Clinical tomosynthesis images (stack of tomographic planes) appear very similar to standard 2D mammography, but lesion detectability is strongly improved in the lesion in-focus plane.

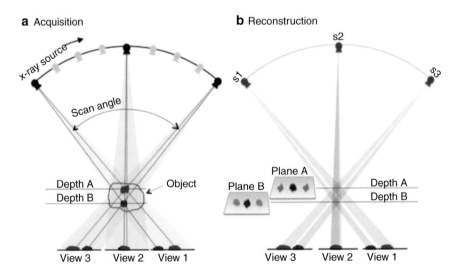

**Fig. 1.1** Tomosynthesis acquisition (**a**) and reconstruction (**b**). Only three projections are represented to illustrate the principle, while in real systems the number of projections ranges between 9 and 25 (From Reiser et al. 2014)

In the following, the details of acquisition and reconstruction will be explored, to better figure out the contribution of each physical/technological factor to DBT images.

## 1.2 Acquisition in Tomosynthesis

There are five digital breast tomosynthesis systems currently available in the European market, three of them received the FDA approval and are available also in the United States. All those systems can perform both standard mammography and tomosynthesis.

In Table 1.1 is reported a summary of the main physical parameters illustrating the differences across manufacturers for each DBT solution (Sechopoulos 2013a, part I).

### 1.2.1 Anode/Filter Material and Technique Factors

It can be noticed from Table 1.1 that the DBT systems mostly use tungsten (W) anode with silver (Ag) or rhodium (Rh) or aluminum (Al) filter, in order to obtain more penetrating X-ray beams than those used for 2D mammography. The only exception is GE, adopting mainly the Rh/Rh in DBT acquisition. Kilovoltage is usually higher than values used for mammography acquisition. The reason why in DBT X-ray beams with higher photon energy are used versus mammography is that the

**Table 1.1** Physical characteristics of the five commercial solutions for digital breast tomosynthesis

| Manufacturer | Fuji | GE | Hologic | IMS | Siemens |
|---|---|---|---|---|---|
| Anode material | W | Mo or Rh | W | W | W |
| Filter material | Al or Rh | Mo or Rh | Ag | Ag | Rh |
| Detector | a-Se FPD | CsI FPD | a-Se FPD | a-Se FPD | a-Se FPD |
| Pixel size ($\mu$m) | 150/100 (ST mode) 100/50 (HR mode) | 100 | 140* (*70 rebinned) | 85 | 85 |
| Pixel shape | Hexagonal | Square | Square | Square | Square |
| Tube motion | Continuous | Step-and-shoot | Continuous | Step-and-shoot | Continuous |
| Sweep angle (°) | 15 (ST mode) 40 (HR mode) | 25 | 15 | 40 | 50 |
| N° of projections | 15 | 9 | 15 | 13 | 25 |
| Dose/projection | Uniform | Uniform | Uniform | Variable | Uniform |
| Antiscatter grid | No | Yes | No | No | No |

inherent contrast of the series if low-dose projections is not very important (as it was in mammography) because the benefit of tomosynthesis derives from its capability of improving lesion conspicuity by reducing the anatomical noise (Yaffe et al. 2014).

### 1.2.2 Detector Type and In-plane Resolution

All the commercial systems mount a flat panel detector (FPD), either with a scintillator (cesium iodide) or a photoconductor (selenium) to convert X-rays in a different type of signal. In the GE system, the X-ray photons entering the panel interact with the cesium iodide (CsI) layer, and are converted in light photons, which constitute the signal collected by the flat panel. In all the other systems, the X-ray photons create electric charges in the selenium layer, and a strong electric field drags those charges to the FPD. Each system uses the same flat panel for both mammography and tomosynthesis acquisition.

The original pixel size of the FPD used in mammography is 50 μm for Fuji, 70 μm for Hologic, 85 μm for IMS and Siemens, and 100 μm for GE. In tomosynthesis, GE, IMS, and Siemens use the same pixel size, Hologic opts for $2 \times 2$ pixel rebinning with an effective pixel size of 140 μm, and Fuji proposes a hexagonal pixel with the opportunity of modulating the effective pixel size from 50 μm up to 150 μm.

As the detector pixel size is either the same or comparable with that used for mammography acquisition, the in-plane resolution ($x$-$y$) of tomosynthesis images (tomographic planes) is high, very close to the resolution of mammography images.

### 1.2.3 Tube Motion

The tube motion around the breast can be either continuous or step-and-shoot. The continuous motion is the same used by computer tomography (CT) systems: the X-ray tube moves continuously along the arc, and at given positions, an X-ray pulse is emitted and a low-dose projection acquired. Its major advantage is the acquisition speed, provided that the detector readout is fast enough, while a disadvantage of the continuous motion is the focal spot blur during tube travel. In the step-and-shoot approach, the X-ray tube stops at each position before acquiring each low-dose projection. This avoids the focal spot blur but requires some extra seconds for the overall scan.

For both continuous and step-and-shoot motions, knowledge of the precise angular position each exposure has been performed is necessary, and this information, recorded in the image header, is used by the algorithm to recombine the projection images and reconstruct the breast volume.

Three out of five commercial DBT systems use the continuous tube motion (Fuji, Hologic, Siemens), the remaining two systems (GE and IMS) adopt the step-and-shoot approach.

## 1.2.4   Acquisition Geometry

All the DBT systems currently available work in partial isocentric geometry, with the detector stationary during acquisition and the X-ray source moving in an arc around the compressed breast. Only the Hologic system tilts the image detector to follow the X-ray tube.

An alternative would be offered by full isocentric geometry, in which detector and X-ray source move synchronously around the imaged object. This is the acquisition geometry of CT.

## 1.2.5   Sweep Angle and Number of Projections

The two parameters that characterize tomosynthesis systems are the sweep angle (or scan angle), i.e., the whole arc traveled by the gantry from first to last projection acquisition, and the number of projections (Roth et al. 2014). As reported in Table 1.1, commercial systems are very different in this respect. The sweep angle ranges from a minimum of 15° (±7.5°) for the Hologic equipment and a maximum of 50° (±25°) for the Siemens system. The Fuji product provides two alternative settings, one called "standard mode" equivalent to the Hologic solution and a second one called "high-resolution mode," with a wider scan angle (40°). The GE system works with an intermediate arc of 25° (±12.5°). The number of low-dose projection ranges from a minimum of 9 (GE) to a maximum of 25 (Siemens).

In general, small scan angles are better for "in-plane resolution" and small objects like microcalcifications are better depicted, while wide angles improve the "out-of-plane resolution" (or z-resolution), and this is preferable for large objects, like masses, whose representation is not limited to an individual in-focus plane. However, the general principle of maximizing the angular range in tomosynthesis is not applicable because of the stationarity of the detector determining a reduction of the effective field of view (FOV) when projections are taken at wide angles. Moreover, due to the constraint applied by manufacturers to keep the radiation dose for a DBT series not much higher than the dose level for a standard mammography view, the use of a wide sweep angle means an increase of the number of projections and the need to decrease the exposure per projection, which should be limited by the presence of quantum noise.

DBT systems mostly distribute radiation dose uniformly along the scan angle, i.e., the same product current x time (mAs) is used for each projection. The only exception is the IMS solution, which uses about 50 % of the total dose for the central projection (to obtain a quasi-standard mammogram), while the remaining dose is variably distributed along the scan angle, with angled projections obtained with a variable angular sampling.

## 1.2.6   Scatter Radiation

Scatter radiation is known to degrade image quality in standard 2D mammography. For this reason, the use of antiscatter grids has been introduced. Grids are constituted of lead septs oriented in the cathode-anode direction and focused toward the X-ray source; the role of the lead septs is to absorb scattered photons and leave unchanged the trajectory of primary photons. However, the grid usage has also determined the need of increasing radiation dose because the grid lines absorb preferably but not exclusively scattered photons. Despite this side effect on radiation dose, grids are systematically used in mammography because they strongly improve image quality, especially for thick breasts.

In tomosynthesis scatter radiation is still present, but most manufacturers chose to not use an antiscatter grid for multiple reasons: the first is that conventional grids cannot be used as they are out of focus for any projection acquired with the X-ray source at a different angle than 0° and the second is that scatter radiation mainly degrades image contrast, but, as stated for the technique factors, the strong point of tomosynthesis is its capability in reducing the anatomical noise, and consequently, the contrast of the projection images becomes a secondary factor. Finally, it should be noticed that the will of keeping radiation dose per DBT projection as low as possible means that such dose level must be set to produce a sufficient signal-to-noise ratio in the projection image; also the scattered photons contribute to the signal-to-noise ratio and, as such, may have some positive effects on DBT quality.

The only manufacturer who still uses a grid in tomosynthesis is GE that developed a special grid with the lead septa oriented parallel to the chest wall in order to capture the scattered photons while maintaining grid focus during acquisition. As for standard mammography, the benefit of grid use is more evident for thick breasts, for which the amount of scattered radiation is more significant.

## 1.3   Reconstruction in Tomosynthesis

Reconstruction of volumetric information from a limited number of low-dose projections acquired within a limited angle is a challenge. In fact, the amount of tomographic information available from acquisition is only partial, and most information necessary for a volumetric reconstruction is missing.

## 1.3.1   Reconstruction Algorithms

Reconstruction algorithms used in tomosynthesis are similar to those used in CT, with some difficulties due to the limited geometry, as mentioned above. There are two main categories, the very classical filtered back-projection (FBP) and the more recent iterative techniques (Sechopoulos 2013b, part II).

Back-projection (BP) just reverses the projection process and realigns structures spatially, obtaining multiple tomographic planes where signal coming from structure belonging to each plane are reinforced (in focus) while any other out-of-plane

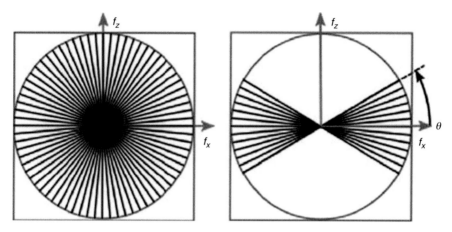

**Fig. 1.2** *Left*: Fourier space coverage in CT acquisition geometry. *Right*: Fourier space coverage in DBT acquisition geometry

structure is blurred. Unfortunately, images reconstructed from pure back-projection are unavoidably blurred, and filtration is required to remove blurring (FBP). This is the reference algorithm used in conventional CT, and its major benefit was to be fast, even in the early days of CT when computers were not as powerful as today. Filtered back-projection is performed in the frequency space, also called Fourier domain. Figure 1.2 compares the information available for reconstruction when a full CT acquisition is performed (left: full angular coverage, many projections) to the limited information available when a DBT acquisition is performed (right, limited angle, limited number of projections). Because of the very poor geometrical sampling of tomosynthesis acquisition, the spatial resolution in the direction perpendicular to the detector plane ($z$-direction) is very limited (Wu et al. 2003).

The iterative techniques include both algebraic and statistical algorithms. They take advantage from the improved performance of computing systems. The iterative reconstruction, currently implemented also in computed tomography, shows particular benefits in tomosynthesis because they can face better than FBP the limitations on image quality caused by the geometrical limitations. Iterative algorithms produce tomographic images with good sharpness and high signal-to-noise ratio. Moreover, they are effective in reducing the reconstruction artifacts caused by the spatial undersampling of tomosynthesis acquisition (Wu et al. 2004).

### 1.3.2   Reconstructed "Objects"

Three different types of "objects" are reconstructed in tomosynthesis:

1. Tomographic planes (mostly called "slices")
2. Slabs
3. 2D synthetic views

As tomosynthesis is often considered a "small angle CT," the CT language has been adopted for tomosynthesis. The main reconstructed object is a stack of tomographic planes, i.e., a set of images reproducing the content of planes at different depths in the breast obtained by reconstructing the breast volume and sampling the tomographic planes with a certain sampling interval. Tomosynthesis review is usually performed by scrolling the tomographic planes in the depth direction manually or through a cine-loop mode.

The term "slice" used to indicate a CT-reconstructed image representing the content of a body section cannot be applied with the same meaning in tomosynthesis. In fact, in CT acquisition the detector array is oriented in the $z$-direction of the patient, and a parameter called "slice thickness" is set before the CT acquisition starts; it determines the thickness of the body section represented by each reconstructed image and thereby the resolution in $z$-direction. In other words, a reconstructed image in CT includes information coming from a section of the patient and, as such, has a thickness. Tomosynthesis setup is different: the image detector is planar, and the tomographic scan acquires a certain number of projection images; the information in $z$-direction is not directly acquired but is derived from the volumetric reconstruction. The algorithm produces a set of planes parallel to the detector plane, spaced by 0.5–1.0 mm one to each other. In other words, tomosynthesis images are not slices (plane thickness is zero), but planes and what is usually reported as "slice thickness" is actually the distance between adjacent planes. Distance between planes is 1 mm for four out of five systems considered in Table 1.1. Only GE system uses a sampling interval of 0.5 mm. The sampling interval, together with the breast compressed thickness, determines the number of reconstructed planes. A 5 cm breast reconstructed by DBT at 1 mm includes a stack of 50 images. As reconstructed planes have the same weight (in bits) of standard mammography views, the overall weight of a DBT exam is definitely higher. For the 5 cm breast considered above, the standard four views (two CCs plus two MLOs) of a bilateral mammography can weigh between 60 and 200 MB, while four views of a bilateral tomosynthesis weigh from 3 GB up to 10 GB.

Other types of images which can be reconstructed from tomosynthesis are "slabs", i.e., "thick slices" obtained by adding together a certain number of tomographic planes. Slabs have thickness, typically 1 cm or more, and are particularly useful to detect microcalcification clusters. In fact, microcalcifications usually grouped in clusters in 2D mammography may be sparse along the depth in the tomographic reconstruction and lose their cluster aspect. Furthermore, slabs allow a quick review of the breast volume, before getting into the details of the tomographic planes if some type of potentially pathological feature is detected. The reviewing workflow is one of the open questions of tomosynthesis, especially when "high-rate" environment are counted, as breast cancer screening, and slabs seem a way to dramatically reduce the radiologists' interpretation time.

Finally, the last "reconstructed objects" derived from tomosynthesis are the "synthetic 2D mammograms." It is a pseudo-mammography, conceptually obtainable by collapsing the breast reconstructed volume onto a plane. Compared to standard 2D mammography views, synthetic 2D views are obtained at zero radiation dose. Moreover, as synthetic views come from DBT reconstructions, they include the major benefit of tomosynthesis, i.e., the reduction of the anatomical noise, increasing lesion conspicuity.

## 1.4    Radiation Dose

Radiation dose in tomosynthesis is evaluated by the mean (or average) glandular dose, MGD, the same parameter used in mammography. It is calculated applying conversion factors computed by Monte Carlo technique to the entrance-measured dose. Compared to mammography MGD, the calculation of MGD with tomosynthesis includes an angular dependence.

In general, the radiation dose level for the acquisition of a tomosynthesis series (associated to a breast view) is expected to be higher than the dose level used to obtain a standard digital mammogram (Svahn et al. 2015). In fact, despite the dose per projection is kept low, in tomosynthesis multiple projection images (between 9 and 25 with current systems) are necessary to permit the volumetric reconstruction, and this unavoidably leads to a dose increase. Most of data come from studies using prototype systems, for which radiation dose for one DBT view was often set "equivalent" to the dose used for 2-view mammography. There are very few results available from the literature about tomosynthesis radiation dose for commercial systems. Depending on the system, its number of projections, X-ray tube, automatic exposure control design, the ratio between the dose per breast tomosynthesis view (CC, MLO, etc.), and the dose per mammography view are usually between 1 and 2 (Feng and Sechopoulos 2012).

However, the reason why there is a certain concern about the increased exposure to radiation dose due to tomosynthesis is associated to the clinical protocol mostly used in screening trials with tomosynthesis. Such protocol includes standard mammography in two views and tomosynthesis in two views, and almost all the results published show the improved clinical performance of the combination of mammography and tomosynthesis compared to mammography alone. With this protocol, also assuming that manufacturers will optimize systems to make dose in DBT equal to dose in mammography, radiation dose would be systematically doubled because of the double examination, and this is questionable in the light of radiation protection, especially in screening population.

The introduction of synthetic 2D mammograms and the positive results obtained indicate that in the next future synthetic mammography obtained from tomosynthesis will replace standard mammography, which will become unnecessary. In other words, the concern about the increased dose level by tomosynthesis can be significantly reappraised if the perspective is to acquire tomosynthesis alone and derive synthetic mammography, at zero dose, from the reconstruction process (Skaane et al. 2014).

# References

Burgess AE, Jacobson FL, Judy PF (2001) Human observer detection experiments with mammograms and power-law noise. Med Phys 28:419–437

Feng SS, Sechopoulos I (2012) Clinical digital breast tomosynthesis system: dosimetric characterization. Radiology 263:35–42

Niklason LT, Christian BT, Niklason LE, Kopans DB, Castleberry DE, Opsahl-Ong BH, Landberg CE, Slanetz PJ, Giardino AA, Moore R, Albagli D, DeJule MC, Fitzgerald PF, Fobare DF, Giambattista BW, Kwasnick RF, Liu J, Lubowski SJ, Possin GE, Richotte JF, Wei CY, Wirth RF (1997) Digital tomosynthesis in breast imaging. Radiology 205:399–406

Park JM, Franken EA Jr, Garg M, Fajardo LL, Niklason LT (2007) Breast tomosynthesis: present considerations and future applications. Radiographics 27(Suppl 1):S231–S240

Reiser I, Sechopoulos I (2014) A review of digital breast tomosynthesis. Med Phys Int 2:57–66

Roth RG, Maidment AD, Weinstein SP, Roth SO, Conant EF (2014) Digital breast tomosynthesis: lessons learned from early clinical implementation. Radiographics 34:E89–E102

Sechopoulos I (2013a) A review of breast tomosynthesis. Part I. The image acquisition process. Med Phys 40:014301

Sechopoulos I (2013b) A review of breast tomosynthesis. Part II. Image reconstruction, processing and analysis, and advanced applications. Med Phys 40:014302

Skaane P, Bandos AI, Eben EB, Jebsen IN, Krager M, Haakenaasen U, Ekseth U, Izadi M, Hofvind S, Gullien R (2014) Two-view digital breast tomosynthesis screening with synthetically reconstructed projection images: comparison with digital breast tomosynthesis with full-field digital mammographic images. Radiology 271:655–663

Svahn TM, Houssami N, Sechopoulos I, Mattsson S (2015) Review of radiation dose estimates in digital breast tomosynthesis relative to those in two-view full-field digital mammography. Breast 24:93–99

Wu T, Stewart A, Stanton M, McCauley T, Phillips W, Kopans DB, Moore RH, Eberhard JW, Opsahl-Ong B, Niklason L, Williams MB (2003) Tomographic mammography using a limited number of low-dose cone-beam projection images. Med Phys 30:365–380

Wu T, Moore RH, Rafferty EA, Kopans DB (2004) A comparison of reconstruction algorithms for breast tomosynthesis. Med Phys 31:2636–2647

Yaffe MJ, Mainprize JG (2014) Digital tomosynthesis: technique. Radiol Clin North Am 52:489–497

# Breast Cancer Screening with Digital Breast Tomosynthesis

**2**

Per Skaane

## 2.1    Introduction

Mammography screening has proven effective in reducing mortality from breast cancer due to early diagnosis of small preclinical and node-negative breast cancers. The use of screening mammography is based on the assumption that breast cancer is a progressive disease, and early detection will have an improved prognosis. The implementation of organized population-based screening programs in many Western countries is based on the mortality reduction shown in the randomized controlled trials (RCT). The first RCT carried out in the state of New York in the 1960s as well as the following RCTs in the 1970s and 1980s all used screen-film mammography (SFM). The image quality of SFM in some of these trials was rather poor as compared with present standard. The image quality of SFM improved very much at the end of the last century. Image quality was further improved with full-field digital mammography (FFDM) which was implemented in breast cancer screening at the beginning of this century. FFDM offers several benefits in organized screening programs: reduction of technical failure recalls; reduction of glandular dose; higher work flow; simplified archival, retrieval, and transmission of images; simpler implementation of computer-aided detection (CAD); and the potential for telemammography and screening program reorganizations. An improvement using FFDM was found especially in women with dense breast parenchyma and for the detection of DCIS manifesting as fine microcalcifications in women with dense breasts (Pisano et al. 2005; Skaane 2009).

Conventional mammography, SFM as well as FFDM, has two serious inherent limitations: a low sensitivity (cancer detection rate) in women with dense breast parenchyma and a low specificity (false-positive interpretations) causing unnecessary

P. Skaane
Department of Radiology, Oslo University Hospital Ullevaal, University of Oslo,
Kirkeveien 166, Oslo 0407, Norway
e-mail: PERSKA@ous-hf.no

© Springer International Publishing Switzerland 2016
A. Tagliafico et al. (eds.), *Digital Breast Tomosynthesis: A Practical Approach*,
DOI 10.1007/978-3-319-28631-0_2

11

recalls. The reason for low sensitivity is the masking effect of overlying breast parenchyma; the noncalcified breast cancer is obscured and missed by the reader. The reason for the false positives is that summation of normal breast parenchyma on conventional mammography occasionally may simulate a cancer. The consequence is that the woman must be recalled for assessment to exclude the presence of a mass.

Consequently, there is a need for improvement in the mammographic technique used in breast cancer screening.

## 2.2    Potential Advances of Tomosynthesis in Screening

Digital breast tomosynthesis (DBT) is based on a full-field digital mammography (FFDM) platform. It was more than 15 years ago that this technique was presented as having the potential to improve the specificity as well as the early detection of breast cancer (Niklason et al. 1997). For tomosynthesis acquisition, the x-ray tube moves through a proscribed arc, and several low-dose projection images are acquired. DBT images are obtained in the same standard projections (craniocaudal, CC, and mediolateral oblique, MLO) as conventional screening mammography. The arc of movement and the number of exposures vary among manufacturers. Tomosynthesis is often called "3D" mammography, but it is important to keep in mind that DBT is only a quasi-3D examination due to the limited angle of scanning. Images are reconstructed into a stack of 1 mm slices. Tomosynthesis reduces the obscuring effect of overlying and underlying breast tissue.

Elimination of superimposed breast tissue using tomosynthesis should improve the detection of lesions otherwise hidden by the dense parenchyma. Consequently, DBT may identify cancers not detectable on 2D images (Fig. 2.1) and thus increase the sensitivity (cancer detection rate) in mammography screening. The cancer visibility on DBT is significantly superior to FFDM (Andersson et al. 2008). Initially, there was much discussion whether one-view or two-view DBT should have the potential to replace two-view FFDM (Gennaro et al. 2013; Svahn et al. 2010). This issue should partly be viewed in a historical perspective: Some vendors did not have DBT equipment suitable for high-volume screening, and there was much concern about the increased radiation dose when implementing tomosynthesis. A summary analysis of studies showed, however, that the most consistent effect of improvement in breast cancer detection was seen in studies using two-view DBT with FFDM (Svahn and Houssami 2015). An interesting study compared the cancer visibility on DBT CC view versus DBT MLO view and reported that only just over half (54 %) of cancers were equally seen on both views, 7 % were only seen on one view, and a significantly larger number of cancers (35 %) were either better or only seen on the CC view (Beck et al. 2013).

Furthermore, tomosynthesis has the potential to improve lesion interpretation and to reduce the number of false-positive interpretations caused by superimposed breast tissue. The specificity in mammography screening would consequently be improved, and the recall rates decreased. Of special importance for breast cancer screening is the fact that DBT can replace conventional supplemental views

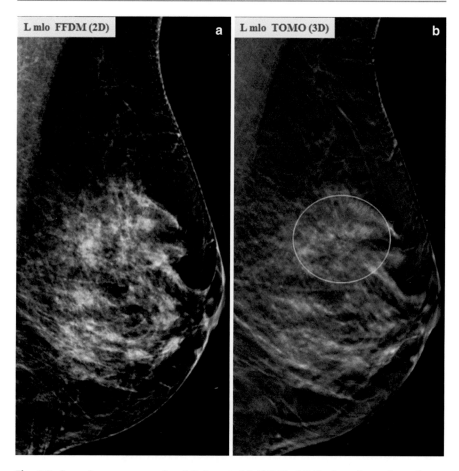

**Fig. 2.1** Screening mammography, left breast. (**a**) FFDM. MLO view shows dense breast parenchyma but no abnormality. Both independent readers for 2D only had a normal score. (**b**) Tomosynthesis demonstrates architectural distortion. Both independent readers gave a true positive score. Histology revealed radial scar with DCIS G3, 11 mm

(Fig. 2.2) for the evaluation of noncalcified findings recalled from screening (Brandt et al. 2013). An experimental clinical study reported a 30 % reduction in recall rate for cancer-free examinations that would otherwise have led to recall if FFDM had been used alone (Gur et al. 2009). Thus, DBT may be an alternative to supplemental mammographic views for noncalcified lesions (Hakim et al. 2010; Noroozian et al. 2012; Tagliafico et al. 2012; Zuley et al. 2013). Consequently, so-called pseudo-lesions due to superimposed breast tissue can be "downgraded" at screening inter-pretation or, where double reading is used, at consensus or arbitration meeting, reducing the need for a callback.

In summary, addition of tomosynthesis to FFDM offers the potential dual benefit of significantly increased sensitivity (cancer detection rate) and significantly reduced recall rates in a breast cancer screening programs (Michell et al. 2012; Rafferty et al. 2013).

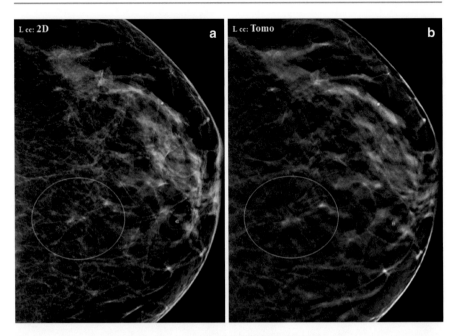

**Fig. 2.2** Screening mammography, left breast. (**a**) FFDM. CC view of the left breast shows a nonspecific asymmetric density in the posteromedial part of the breast. At assessment due to the DBT finding, the adjunct FFDM cone-magnification views did not demonstrate any definite abnormality. (**b**) Tomosynthesis shows a desmoplastic reaction with long thin spiculae suspicious of malignancy. Histology revealed invasive ductal carcinoma G2, 4.5 mm

## 2.3    Tomosynthesis in Breast Cancer Screening

Considering the promising results from experimental clinical studies on tomosynthesis, it was only a question of time when the first studies on DBT in breast cancer screening would be started. However, there were some problems and challenges before studies on DBT in the screening setting could be rolled out. Tomosynthesis received the US Food and Drug Administration approval as late as 2011. The screening studies published from the USA have so far been retrospective studies in which facilities implementing DBT in a screening setting usually have used historical control groups for comparison. In the European countries, there has been no formal approval of the technology for screening, and the potential increased radiation dose to healthy women has been a concern.

Finally, several retrospective US studies and three prospective European trials on DBT in mammography screening have been carried out so far. There are important differences between mammography screening in the US and the European countries, and it is reasonable to discuss the US and the European studies separately.

## 2.3.1 Retrospective US Screening Studies

The retrospective US studies on tomosynthesis in mammography screening published so far are summarized in Table 2.1. In most studies more than one radiological site was involved, and consequently the number of examinations from each institution was occasionally rather small. In some studies the populations are rather heterogeneous and include women with a personal history of breast cancer (Destounis et al. 2014) and thus are very different from the population-based European programs. Another study, however, reported no significant differences regarding age, family history of breast cancer, history of hormone use, or whether

**Table 2.1** Retrospective US studies on DBT in breast cancer screening published so far

| Study (author/ place) | Year (publ) | Population | | Recall rate | | | Cancer detection | | |
|---|---|---|---|---|---|---|---|---|---|
| | | | *n* | | % | Sign. | | % | Sign. |
| Destounis S, Rochester, NY[a] | 2014 | FFDM: | 524 | FFDM: | 11.5 | | FFDM: | 0.38 | |
| | | DBT: | 524 | DBT: | 4.2 | Sign. | DBT: | 0.57 | n.a. |
| Durand MA, Yale, CT[b] | 2015 | FFDM: | 9364 | FFDM: | 12.3 | | FFDM: | 0.57 | |
| | | DBT: | 8591 | DBT: | 7.8 | Sign. | DBT: | 0.59 | n.s. |
| Greenberg JS, Potomac, MD[c] | 2014 | FFDM: | 38,674 | FFDM: | 16.2 | | FFDM: | 0.49 | |
| | | DBT: | 20,943 | DBT: | 13.6 | Sign. | DBT: | 0.63 | Sign. |
| Haas BM, Yale, CT[d] | 2013 | FFDM: | 7058 | FFDM: | 12.0 | | FFDM: | 0.52 | |
| | | DBT: | 6100 | DBT: | 8.4 | Sign. | DBT: | 0.57 | n.s. |
| Lourenco AP, Providence, RI[e] | 2015 | FFDM: | 12,577 | FFDM: | 9.3 | | FFDM: | 0.54 | |
| | | DBT: | 12,921 | DBT: | 6.4 | Sign. | DBT: | 0.46 | n.s. |
| McCarthy AM, Philadelphia, PA[f] | 2014 | FFDM: | 10,728 | FFDM: | 10.4 | | FFDM: | 0.46 | |
| | | DBT: | 15,571 | DBT: | 8.8 | Sign. | DBT: | 0.55 | n.s. |
| Rose SL, Houston, TX[g] | 2013 | FFDM: | 13,856 | FFDM: | 8.7 | | FFDM: | 0.40 | |
| | | DBT: | 9499 | DBT: | 5.5 | Sign. | DBT: | 0.54 | n.s. |
| Friedewald SM, Park Ridge, IL | 2014 | FFDM: | 281,187 | FFDM: | 10.7 | | FFDM: | 0.42 | |
| | | DBT: | 173,663 | DBT: | 9.1 | Sign. | DBT: | 0.54 | Sign. |

The studies are listed alphabetically according to author (except for the last Friedewald paper which is a pooling of data already published in some of the other studies). Year of publication, number of women included, recall rate with significance, and cancer detection with significance are listed. All studies include single reading for 2D (FFDM) as well as for 3D (FFDM+DBT)
Note: The DBT reading mode includes FFDM plus DBT for all studies
Significance (sign.): conclusion given by the authors (in general $p < 0.05$)
N.a.: no p-value given by the authors
[a]Destounis S et al.: *J Clin Imaging Sci* 2014;4:9
[b]Durand MA et al.: *Radiology* 2015;274:85–92
[c]Greenberg JS et al.: *AJR* 2014;203:1–7
[d]Haas BM et al.: *Radiology* 2013;269:694–700
[e]Lourenco AP et al.: *Radiology* 2015;274:337–342
[f]McCarthy AM et al.: *J Natl Cancer Inst* 2014; doi:10.1093/jnci/dju316
[g]Friedewald SM et al.: *JAMA* 2014;311:2499–2507

the screening study was baseline or subsequent (Greenberg et al. 2014). Experience in breast imaging and training of the readers in the new technique (tomosynthesis) varied as would be expected among the studies and sites (Haas et al. 2013; Lourenco et al. 2015; McCarthy et al. 2014). Some studies included computer-aided detection (CAD) for interpretation of 2D images (Durand et al. 2015; Lourenco et al. 2015). Some studies could not rule out self-selection bias because women elected whether they would undergo the conventional imaging or the new technology (Rose et al. 2013).

The most important finding from the US tomosynthesis screening studies is that all studies demonstrated a significant decrease in the recall rate (Table 2.1). However, it should be noted that the recall rates are quite different from the European screening programs. One might also expect significant reduction in the recall rate in European countries but not as dramatic as observed in US studies since many European organized screening programs have a recall rate below 3 % according to the European guidelines. More problematic to interpret are the different results regarding the cancer detection rates in the US studies (Table 2.1). All but one of the US studies reported an increase in the cancer detection rate using DBT, but the improvement was statistically significant in only two of the studies (Table 2.1). The explanation for nonsignificant values is probably the small number of cancers in some studies. It is noticeable that one study even reported a lower cancer detection rate using DBT (Lourenco et al. 2015); however, that was not statistically significant and could be due to chance.

It should be kept in mind that all the US studies published so far have used two view (CC and MLO) for 2D as well as for 3D examinations and they have all been carried out with equipment from the same manufacturer (Selenia Dimension, Hologic).

The large US study pooling the results from 13 academic and nonacademic breast centers is of much important (Friedewald et al. 2014). The study populations are huge, including a total of 281,187 women undergoing FFDM only and 173,663 women having FFDM plus DBT. As would be expected, there was a considerable variation among the different sites. The model-adjusted recall rate was 10.7 % (95 % CI, 8.9–12.4) and 9.1 % (95 % CI, 7.3–10.8) and the cancer detection rate 0.42 % (95 % CI, 0.38–0.47) and 0.54 % (95 % CI, 0.49–0.60) for FFDM and FFDM plus DBT, respectively. Of interest is the increased detection from DBT in this study, approaching estimates reported from the European studies.

## 2.3.2   Prospective European Screening Studies

Three prospective European trials on tomosynthesis in breast cancer screening have been published so far, and all of these studies have included women attending an organized screening program. One study (the Italian "Screening with Tomo OR standard Mammo," STORM, carried out in Trento and Verona) has published the final results (Ciatto et al. 2013). From the two other trials, the Norwegian "Oslo Tomosynthesis Screening Trial" OTST and the Swedish "Malmø Breast

Tomosynthesis Screening Trial" MBTST), only interim analyses have been published so far (Skaane et al. 2013a, b; Lång et al. 2015). These three prospective European studies are very different in study design, and this fact must be kept in mind when comparing the results. The three European studies are summarized in Table 2.2. The study design of the three trials might be somewhat difficult to understand unless the papers are read carefully.

The first published study, the Italian STORM trial, examined 7292 women with a median age of 58 years attending a population-based screening program (Ciatto et al. 2013). The study design included a paired sequential reading in two sequential phases, first 2D and then integrated 2D and 3D. The eight readers were breast radiologists with a mean of 8 years experience in mammography screening. The authors concluded that if a conditional recall rule is applied, DBT can show a reduction of 17 % in recalls (Table 2.3). The cancer detection rate increased from 5.3 cancers per 1000 screen using 2D to 8.1 cancers per 1000 screens using integrated 2D plus 3D, i.e., a remarkable increase in the invasive cancer detection rate. Of interest is their finding that the incremental cancer detection was much the same in women with low-density versus high-density parenchyma, although the investigators noted that there was a small number of screening participants classified as having dense breasts. The mean tumor size was 13.5 mm for cancers detected only with 2D + 3D (Ciatto et al. 2013).

The two other larger prospective European trials have so far only published interim analyses. Three publications have been presented from the Norwegian OTST. The Oslo trial is part of the Norwegian Breast Cancer Screening Program (NBCSP) inviting women aged 50–69 years biannually to two-view mammography. The OTST was scheduled for one screening round, i.e., 2 years. The program includes independent double reading with consensus or arbitration before final

**Table 2.2** Prospective European trials comparing full-field digital mammography (FFDM) and digital breast tomosynthesis (DBT) in organized breast cancer screening programs

| Study place | Study period | Population (n) | Age group (years) | Study design | Exam mode | Reading mode |
|---|---|---|---|---|---|---|
| STORM Trento/Verona[a] | 08/2011– 06/2012 | 7292 | >48 | Prospective; paired | 2D: two-view 3D: two-view | Double; sequential |
| OTST Oslo[b] | 11/2010– 12/2012 | 25,547 | 50–69 | Prospective; paired | 2D: two-view 3D: two-view | Double; independent |
| MBTST Malmö[c] | 01/2010– 12/2012 | 15,000 | 40–74 | Prospective; paired | 2D: two-view 3D: one-view | Double; sequential |

The number of women (population) is the final number for the STORM trial (as presented in Table 2.3), the final number of women having tomosynthesis in the OTST trial (but not the number presented in the interim analysis in Table 2.3), and the scheduled number of women in the MBTST (and not the number presented in the interim analysis in Table 2.3)

[a]Screening with Tomo OR standard Mammo STORM: Ciatto S et al.: *Lancet Oncol*, 2013

[b]Oslo Tomosynthesis Screening Trial OTST: Skaane P et al.: *Eur Radiol* 2013

[c]Malmö Breast Tomosynthesis Screening Trial MBTST: Lång K et al. *Eur Radiol* 2015

**Table 2.3** Summary results from the three prospective European tomosynthesis screening studies

| Study | Recall or False Positive change (%) | Cancer detection (n/1000) | All cancer increase (%) | Invasive cancer increase (%) |
|---|---|---|---|---|
| *STORM* Trento/Verona[a] | −17 | FFDM: *5.3* DBT: *8.1 (+2.8)* | +53 | +49 |
| *OTST* Oslo[b] | −13 | FFDM: *6.1* DBT: *8.0 (+1.9)* | +27 | +45 |
| *MBTST* Malmø[c] | +43 | FFDM: *6.3* DBT: *8.9 (+2.6)* | +43 | +42 |
| *US study* Friedewald S[d] | −16 | FFDM: *4.2* DBT *5.4 (+1.2)* | +29 | +41 |

The retrospective US study with pooled data from other studies is listed at the bottom for comparison. The relative change in recall rate, the cancer detection, and the relative increase in all cancer and for invasive cancer are presented

Note:

[a]Screening with Tomo OR standard Mammo STORM: Ciatto S et al.: *Lancet Oncol*, 2013

   The decreased recall change is "estimated conditional recall"

[b]Oslo Tomosynthesis Screening Trial OTST: Skaane P et al.: *Radiology* 2013

   The decreased number of false positive scores and not actual callbacks are presented

[c]Malmø Breast Tomosynthesis Screening Trial MBTST: Lång K et al. *Eur Radiol* 2015

   The increased cancer value is based on one-view DBT

[d]Friedewald SM et al.: *JAMA* 2014

   Numbers for the 13 sites are model adjusted; range of recall −42 % to +18; range of cancers/1000 was +3.7 to −1.5

decision for recall. Eight radiologists participated in the study, alternating interpretation in the four arms. Batch reading was carried out on one of four dedicated work stations, one for each arm, thus offering absolute independent reading in the four arms. There was a common arbitration meeting for all four arms before decision to recall or not.

- The first analysis from the OTST compared the results of the first year in arm A (FFDM without using CAD) and arm C (FFDM without synthetic 2D images + DBT), including a total of 12,631 paired examinations (Skaane et al. 2013a, b). This study showed a reduction in pre-arbitration false-positive scores of 15 % adjusted for reader ($p < 0.001$) and an increase in the cancer detection rate from 6.1 to 8.0 per 1000 examinations using 2D + 3D as compared with FFDM only (Table 2.3). The second interim analysis published in European Radiology compared independent double reading with 2D and independent double reading with 2D + 3D. The results were similar to those published in the first interim analysis, with a significant reduction in pre-arbitration false-positive scores and a significant increase in the cancer detection rate (Table 2.3). The reduction in pre-arbitration false-positive scores and the increased number of FP recall post-arbitration will hopefully be further analyzed in the final report from this study. The increase in cancer detection was mainly caused by invasive tumors manifesting as spiculated mass and architectural distortion (Fig. 2.3), and there was no increase in DCIS using combined

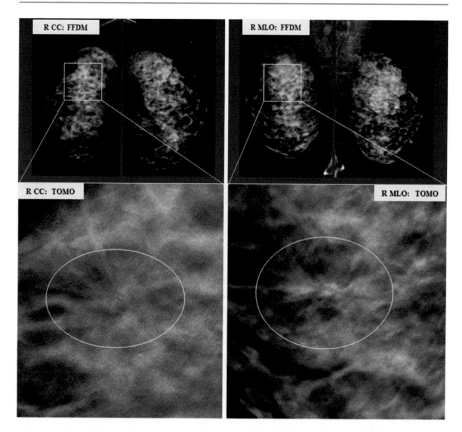

**Fig. 2.3** Screening mammography. The mammographic finding on conventional FFDM (*top, small images*) was a normal score for both breasts by both independent readers. Tomosynthesis (*lower magnification images*) shows a small spiculated mass in the dense breast parenchyma. Histology revealed invasive ductal carcinoma G1 + DCIS G3 (total extent 14 mm)

reading (Skaane et al. 2013a, b). The third interim analysis compared FFDM + DBT with synthetic 2D + DBT. In this study results using an early version of synthesized 2D images from the first study period were compared with an improved version used in the second period of the OTST (Skaane et al. 2014). An important finding was that in period 2 (with the current new version of the synthesized 2D images), there was no significant difference regarding false-positive scores, cancer detection rate, or positive predictive values in the two arms (Skaane et al. 2014).

The third prospective European study is the Malmø Breast Tomosynthesis Screening Trial (MBTST). Women aged 40–74 years invited to the population-based screening in Malmø were included. A sequential reading mode was used in this one-arm single-institution study investigating the use of one-view DBT alone versus two-view FFDM and a combination of one-view DBT (MLO view) and one-view FFDM (CC view). This study did also show a significant and high increase in the cancer detection rate: The detection rate for one-view DBT was 8.8 per 1000 screens as compared to 6.3 per 1000 screens for two-view FFDM ($p<0.0001$), a relative increase of 43 % (Lång et al. 2015). There was an increase in the recall rate when using stand-alone tomosynthesis relative to FFDM of 43 % (Table 2.3), but the recall rate of 3.8 % using DBT is still low and within the acceptable values as recommended by the European guidelines.

### 2.3.3   Conclusions from the Screening Studies

The recall rate should be significantly reduced when DBT is implemented in breast cancer screening, although this will also vary according to the recall rules used. All the retrospective US studies and two of the three prospective European trials have demonstrated a statistically significant reduction in the recall rate using DBT. Only the Malmø trial showed a remarkable high and significant increase in the recall rate. The reason for the increased callback rate in the Malmø trial is an open question but a matter of concern. This study used a sequential reading design, as was also done in the STORM trial, but only a one-view DBT (MLO only) which is different from all the other studies and is the only study to report on stand-alone DBT which may explain the increased FPs. It might perhaps also be explained by a learning curve, and we have to wait for the final results of the Malmø trial. It should be kept in mind that "clean and straight" values for recall rate could not be given in any of the European trials due to their study design.

The cancer detection rate in mammography screening is significantly improved using tomosynthesis. All the three prospective European studies as well as the large US study (Friedewald et al. 2014) demonstrated a significant increase using DBT (Table 2.3). The nonsignificant increase in several of the other US studies (Table 2.1) is most likely explained by low numbers of cancers and by limited statistical power from the sample sizes of these studies that compare independent groups.

## 2.4   Limitations and Challenges of Tomosynthesis in Screening

Experimental clinical studies and the screening studies mentioned above have shown that tomosynthesis potentially might be the next technique for breast cancer screening. It is, however, important to be aware of some challenges when implementing DBT in organized breast screening programs.

### 2.4.1   Radiation Dose and the Need for Synthetic 2D Images

The radiation dose for one-view DBT is approximately the same as for one-view FFDM (Svahn et al. 2014). Consequently, the combined use of two-view FFDM and two-view DBT in screening would mean a doubling of the radiation dose, and doubling of the radiation dose to healthy women in a population-based screening program would not be acceptable. There has been much discussion whether there is a need for 2D as well as 3D images. Theoretically, one might think that tomosynthesis slices of 1 mm thickness throughout the breast would make 2D images superfluous and that 1 mm DBT slices in one of standard projection would make every abnormality visible so that DBT in the other standard projection would be superfluous. However, radiologists will need 2D images for several reasons: comparison of current exams with prior exams and comparison of right versus left breast. And as mentioned above: Cancers are occasionally more obvious on CC views (Andersson et al. 2008), and cancers are often better and occasionally only seen on one DBT view (Beck et al. 2013). Experience so far favor the combination of two-view 2D with two-view DBT.

The solution to the radiation dose challenge when implementing 2D plus 3D is the use of so-called synthetic 2D images. Synthetic 2D images are created by summing and filtering the stack of reconstructed DBT slices, and the image could in some way be compared with maximum intensity projection image ("MIP"). Thus, synthetic 2D images will need no extra radiation exposure, and consequently a screening examination including two-view 2D combined with two-view DBT will have a radiation dose comparable with the conventional two-view FFDM.

Synthetic 2D images have recently gained high enough quality to be considered an alternative to FFDM in combination with DBT. One prospective screening study showed no significant difference in the false-positive scores, the cancer detection rate, or the positive predictive value between synthetic 2D in combination with tomosynthesis and FFDM plus DBT (Skaane et al. 2014). An experimental clinical study showed that synthetic 2D images even as a stand-alone test are comparable in performance to FFDM (Zuley et al. 2014). However, synthetic 2D images plus DBT are for the time being inferior to both FFDM and FFDM plus DBT for depicting microcalcifications and small DCIS (Gilbert et al. 2015). The image quality of synthetic 2D images will probably improve, and it is reasonable to suggest that synthetic 2D images in the future will replace conventional 2D images in combination with DBT in screening (Fig. 2.4).

### 2.4.2  Microcalcifications

There has been some discussion on DBT and the detection and characterization of microcalcifications. An early study concluded that calcifications can be demonstrated with equal or greater clarity on tomosynthesis as on conventional mammography (Kopans et al. 2011). However, a recent study confirmed that although most microcalcification clusters are scored similarly on FFDM and DBT, a minority was classified differently, and this may have clinical relevance (Tagliafico et al. 2015). Theoretically, merging several 1 mm slices of DBT into "slabs" (of varying thickness) should better demonstrate the three-dimensional clusters. This needs, however, to be confirmed in further studies.

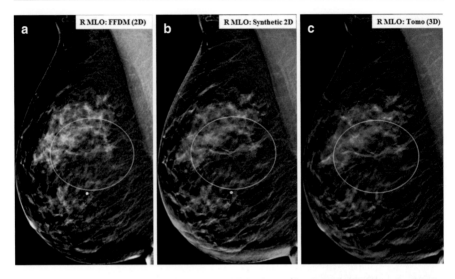

**Fig. 2.4** Screening mammography, right breast MLO views. Histology revealed invasive lobular carcinoma G1, 12 mm. (**a**) FFDM. (**b**) Synthetic 2D image. (**c**) Tomosynthesis. The small mass with large surrounding spiculae is easily seen on synthetic 2D and DBT but is even in retrospect difficult to identify on conventional mammography

There are some interesting aspects regarding microcalcifications, synthetic 2D images, and breast cancer screening. Calcifications are "highlighted" on synthetic 2D images, and this may improve the detection (perception) of fine microcalcifications in women with dense breast parenchyma (Fig. 2.5). However, this highlighting has a price: The analysis (characterization) of some subgroups of microcalcifications may occasionally be insufficient on the synthetic images. In the screening reading session, microcalcifications are often obviously benign, and there is no need for recall, and often they are new and/or highly suspicious, and there is definitely a need for biopsy. Synthetic 2D images in screening will, however, occasionally not allow a decision-making in the reading session or at arbitration meeting, and these cases would need conventional fine-focus magnification views before decision on biopsy and/or for measurement of calcifications extent (Fig. 2.6). This experience is confirmed by recent publications (Gilbert et al. 2015; Tagliafico et al. 2015).

## 2.4.3   Lesions Seen Only on Tomosynthesis

The advantage of tomosynthesis is the detection of small invasive cancers manifesting as spiculated mass or architectural distortion. These cancers are occasionally only seen on DBT and cannot be identified on conventional FFDM even in retrospect (Partyka et al. 2014). Such lesions have a high likelihood of malignancy (Ray et al. 2015). The small spiculated lesions seen only on tomosynthesis may represent a diagnostic challenge, but careful analysis of the DBT exam is important since a reason for nondetection in DBT could also be a lack of experience (Lång et al.

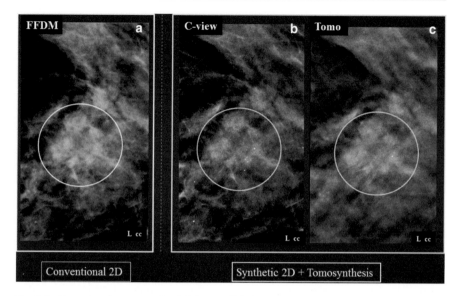

**Fig. 2.5** Screening mammography, left breast, CC views. Histology revealed DCIS 40 mm. (**a**) FFDM. (**b**) Synthetic 2D. (**c**) Tomosynthesis. Note that the microcalcifications are best seen on the synthetic 2D image ("highlighting") and the desmoplastic reaction is seen only on DBT. Both mammographic findings could easily be missed on FFDM. The radiation dose for synthetic 2D+DBT (*right half*) is comparable to conventional FFDM (*left image*)

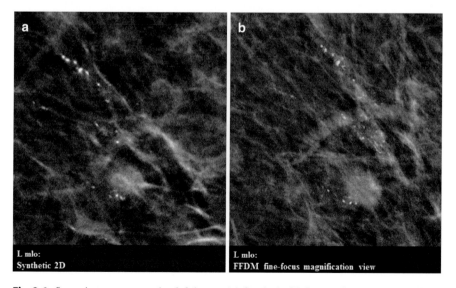

**Fig. 2.6** Screening mammography, left breast. (**a**) Synthetic 2D image shows segmental-linear calcifications highly suspicious for high-grade DCIS. (**b**) FFDM fine-focus magnification image at assessment demonstrates more fine microcalcifications, and the characterization of the calcification is also better. Histology revealed DCIS G3, 30 mm

2014). The reason for missing these small lesions on tomosynthesis, especially if the desmoplastic reaction is not prominent, is most likely a combination of perception and characterization errors.

Tomosynthesis-guided needle biopsy and preoperative needle localization solve most of the problems associated with mammographically and sonographically occult lesions found on DBT. DBT-guided needle procedures are an accurate and fast method, and the clinical performance of DBT-guided vacuum-assisted biopsy is significantly superior to conventional stereotactic vacuum-assisted biopsy (Freer et al. 2015; Schrading et al. 2015).

### 2.4.4  Increased Workload and Interpretation Time

Tomosynthesis is commonly presented on the workstations as a stack of 1 mm thick slices. This means that a breast compressed to a thickness of 5 cm would have 50 slices in one projection. If the breast theoretically would have the same thickness in all four standard views, there would be 200 slices to interpret in addition to the 2D images. It is obvious that the interpretation of tomosynthesis will be more time-consuming. The increased reading time for radiologists might turn out to be one of the really great challenges for implementing DBT in population-based screening program.

The time needed to read 2D plus 3D images varies considerably in the published reports. One experimental clinical study reported a significant increase in mean reading time for 2D + 3D of 77 s as compared with 33 s for 2D only (Bernardi et al. 2012). Another study reported a mean interpretation time of 2.8 min for combined reading as compared with 1.9 min for 2D, which means 47 % longer time (Dang et al. 2014). The reading time for one-view DBT (MLO view only) is of course faster (Lång et al. 2015).

Interpretation time was automatically recorded for all readers in all arms in the OTST. The first interim analysis showed a mean interpretation time of 45 s for 2D only and 91 s for combined 2D + 3D (Skaane et al. 2013a). There is a learning curve effect, and at a later interim analysis, the median reading time was 25 s for 2D and 61 s for 2D plus 3D. Overall, one may conclude that the reading time for combined 2D + 3D interpretation is doubled as compared with 2D only. The additional reading time must be weighted against the significant increase in cancer detection and the reduced callback rates.

## 2.5  The Next Future for Tomosynthesis in Screening

Considering the discussion on pros and cons for mammography screening during the last years, there is no surprise if there is going to be a debate whether DBT is ready for implementation in breast cancer screening or not. The adverse effects of mammography screening including false-positive interpretations, false-negative interpretations and cancers manifesting as interval cancers, and overdiagnosis ("overdetection") have been a hot topic during the last decade. Overdiagnosis is likely to be driven by new technological developments including DBT. What we can conclude already today is that regardless how promising results are presented from ongoing and future studies on tomosynthesis, the "never-ending" controversy on mammography screening will continue.

Tomosynthesis has been considered as "A new era in mammography screening" (Kopans 2014). Several editorials have discussed the implementation of DBT in breast cancer screening. Although DBT represents the most significant improvement in mammography development in recent years and shows extremely promising results, more evidence is needed before a change in well-established mammography screening practice can be more broadly recommended (Houssami and Zackrisson 2013). RCTs assessing the impact of adjunct tomosynthesis on interval cancer rate and other surrogates for aggressive cancer behavior have been suggested (Houssami 2015; Pisano and Yaffe 2014). The IARC working group report (Lauby-Secretan et al. 2015) on breast cancer screening classified the strength of evidence for 2D+DBT regarding increasing detection rate of in situ and invasive cancers as "sufficient," the evidence regarding preferentially increasing the detection of invasive cancers as "limited," and the evidence for reducing the proportion of false-positive screening outcomes as "limited."

Two cost-benefit papers on the value of DBT for screening concluded that there is a clinical and economic favorability of tomosynthesis for screening among commercially insured US women (Bonafede et al. 2015) and that "biennial combined digital mammography and tomosynthesis screening for US women aged 50–74 years with dense breasts is likely to be cost-effective" (Lee et al. 2015).

In conclusion, it must be kept in mind that tomosynthesis is just "a better mammogram." Today, the documentation on benefits of DBT versus FFDM is even better than the evidence when FFDM replaced SFM about a decade ago. Implementation of new modalities like ultrasound or MRI in breast cancer screening for women at average risk would have huge consequences for manpower, be very costly, and need reorganization of existing screening programs. Tomosynthesis would be much easier and more efficient to implement since it is just an improvement of mammography technique and mammography screening is widely implemented on the basis of evidence of screening benefit which could be extended through a more refined form of mammography, tomosynthesis.

# References

Andersson I, Ikeda DM, Zackrisson S et al (2008) Breast tomosynthesis and digital mammography: a comparison of breast cancer visibility and BIRADS classification in a population of cancers with subtle mammographic findings. Eur Radiol 18:2817–2825

Beck N, Butler R, Durand M et al (2013) One-view versus two-view tomosynthesis: a comparison of breast cancer visibility in the mediolateral oblique and craniocaudal views. ARRS Annual Meeting Washington 2013, Scientific session 27. p 177

Bernardi D, Ciatto S, Pellegrini M et al (2012) Application of breast tomosynthesis in screening: incremental effect on mammography acquisition and reading time. Br J Radiol 85:e1174–e1178

Bonafede MM, Kalra VB, Miller JD et al (2015) Value analysis of digital breast tomosynthesis for breast cancer screening in a commercially-insured US population. Clinicoecon Outcomes Res 7:53–63

Brandt KR, Craig DA, Hoskins TL et al (2013) Can digital breast tomosynthesis replace conventional diagnostic mammography views for screening recalls without calcifications? A comparison study in a simulated clinical setting. AJR Am J Roentgenol 200:291–298

Ciatto S, Houssami N, Bernardi D et al (2013) Integration of 3D digital mammography with tomosynthesis for population breast-cancer screening (STORM): a prospective comparison study. Lancet Oncol 14:583–589

Dang PA, Freer PE, Humphrey KL et al (2014) Addition of tomosynthesis to conventional digital mammography: effect on image interpretation time of screening examinations. Radiology 270:49–56

Destounis S, Arieno A, Morgan R (2014) Initial experience with combination digital breast tomosynthesis plus full field digital mammography or full field digital mammography alone in the screening environment. J Clin Imaging Sci 4:9

Durand MA, Haas BM, Yao X et al (2015) Early clinical experience with digital breast tomosynthesis for screening mammography. Radiology 274:85–92

Freer PE, Niell B, Rafferty EA (2015) Preoperative tomosynthesis-guided needle localization of mammographically and sonographically occult breast lesions. Radiology 275:377–383

Friedewald SM, Rafferty EA, Rose SI et al (2014) Breast cancer screening using tomosynthesis in combination with digital mammography. JAMA 311:2499–2507

Gennaro G, Hendrick RE, Ruppel P et al (2013) Performance comparison of single-view digital breast tomosynthesis plus single-view digital mammography with two-view digital mammography. Eur Radiol 23:664–672

Gilbert FJ, Tucker L, Gillan MGC et al (2015) Accuracy of digital breast tomosynthesis for depicting breast cancer subgroups in a UK retrospective reading study (TOMMY trial). Radiology 277:697–706

Greenberg JS, Javitt MC, Katzen J et al (2014) Clinical performance metrics of 3D digital breast tomosynthesis compared with 2D digital mammography for breast cancer screening in community practice. AJR Am J Roentgenol 203:1–7

Gur D, Abrams GS, Chough DM et al (2009) Digital breast tomosynthesis: observer performance study. AJR Am J Roentgenol 193:586–591

Haas BM, Kalra V, Geisel J et al (2013) Comparison of tomosynthesis plus digital mammography and digital mammography alone for breast cancer screening. Radiology 269:694–700

Hakim CM, Chough DM, Ganott MA et al (2010) Digital breast tomosynthesis in the diagnostic environment: a subjective side-by-side review. AJR Am J Roentgenol 195:172–176

Houssami N, Zackrisson S (2013) Digital breast tomosynthesis: the future of mammography screening or much ado about nothing? Expert Rev Med Devices 10:583–585

Houssami N (2015) Digital breast tomosynthesis (3D-mammography) screening: data and implications for population screening. Expert Rev Med Devices 12:377–379. Early online 1–3

Kopans D, Gavenonis S, Halpern E et al (2011) Calcifications in the breast and digital breast tomosynthesis. Breast J 17:638–644

Kopans DB (2014) A new era in mammography screening. Radiology 271:629–631

Lauby-Secretan B, Scoccianti C, Loomis D et al (2015) Breast-cancer screening – viewpoint of the IARC working group. N Engl J Med 372:2353–2358

Lee CI, Cevik M, Alagoz O et al (2015) Comparative effectiveness of combined digital mammography and tomosynthesis screening for women with dense breasts. Radiology 274:772–780

Lourenco AP, Barry-Brooks M, Baird GL et al (2015) Changes in recall type and patient treatment following implementation of screening digital breast tomosynthesis. Radiology 274:337–342

Lång K, Andersson I, Zackrisson S (2014) Breast cancer detection in digital breast tomosynthesis and digital mammography – a side-by-side review of discrepant cases. Br J Radiol. doi:10.1259/bjr.20140080

Lång K, Andersson I, Rosso A et al (2015) Performance of one-view breast tomosynthesis as a stand-alone breast cancer screening modality: results from the Malmø breast tomosynthesis screening trial, a population-based study. Eur Radiol. doi:10.1007/s00330-015-3803-3

McCarthy AM, Kontos D, Synnestvedt M et al (2014) Screening outcomes following implementation of digital breast tomosynthesis in a general-population screening program. J Natl Cancer Inst. doi:10.1093/jnci/dju316

Michell MJ, Iqbal A, Wasan RK et al (2012) A comparison of the accuracy of film-screen mammography, full-field digital mammography, and digital breast tomosynthesis. Clin Radiol 67:976–981

Niklason LT, Christian BT, Niklason LE et al (1997) Digital tomosynthesis in breast imaging. Radiology 205:399–406

Noroozian M, Hadjiiski L, Rahnama-Moghadam S et al (2012) Digital breast tomosynthesis is comparable to mammographic spot views for mass characterization. Radiology 262:61–68

Partyka L, Lourenco AP, Mainiero MB (2014) Detection of mammographically occult architectural distortion on digital breast tomosynthesis screening: Initial clinical experience. AJR Am J Roentgenol 203:216–222

Pisano ED, Gatsonis C, Hendrick E et al (2005) Diagnostic performance of digital versus film mammography for breast cancer screening. N Engl J Med 353:1773–1783

Pisano ED, Yaffe MJ (2014) Breast cancer screening. Should tomosynthesis replace digital mammography? JAMA 311:2488–2489

Rafferty EA, Park JM, Philpotts LE et al (2013) Assessing radiologist performance using combined digital mammography and breast tomosynthesis compared with digital mammography alone: Results of a multicentre, multireader trial. Radiology 266:104–113

Ray KM, Turner E, Sickles EA et al (2015) Suspicious findings at digital breast tomosynthesis occult to conventional digital mammography: imaging features and pathology findings. Breast J. doi:10.1111/tbj.12446

Rose SL, Tidwell AL, Bujnoch LJ et al (2013) Implementation of breast tomosynthesis in a routine screening practice: an observational study. AJR Am J Roentgenol 200:1401–1408

Schrading S, Distelmaier M, Dirrichs T et al (2015) Digital breast tomosynthesis-guided vacuum-assisted breast biopsy: initial experiences and comparison with prone stereotactic vacuum-assisted biopsy. Radiology 274:654–662

Skaane P (2009) Studies comparing screen-film mammography and full-field digital mammography in breast cancer screening: updated review. Acta Radiol 50:3–14

Skaane P, Bandos AI, Gullien R et al (2013a) Comparison of digital mammography alone and digital mammography plus tomosynthesis in a population-based screening program. Radiology 267:47–56

Skaane P, Bandos AI, Gullien R et al (2013b) Prospective trial comparing full-field digital mammography (FFDM) versus combined FFDM and tomosynthesis in a population-based screening programme using independent double reading with arbitration. Eur Radiol 23:2061–2071

Skaane P, Bandos AI, Eben EB et al (2014) Two-view digital breast tomosynthesis screening with synthetically reconstructed projection images: comparison with digital breast tomosynthesis with full-field digital mammographic images. Radiology 271:655–663

Svahn T, Andersson I, Chakraborty D et al (2010) The diagnostic accuracy of dual-view digital mammography, single-view breast tomosynthesis and a dual-view combination of breast tomosynthesis and digital mammography in a free-response observer performance study. Radiat Prot Dosim 139:113–117

Svahn TM, Houssami N, Sechopoulos I et al (2014) Review of radiation dose estimates in digital breast tomosynthesis relative to those in two-view full-field digital mammography. Breast. doi:10.1016/j.breast.2014.12.002

Svahn TM, Houssami N (2015) Digital breast tomosynthesis in one or two views as a replacement or adjunct technique to full-field digital mammography. Radiat Prot Dosim. doi:10.1093/rpd/ncv078

Tagliafico A, Astengo D, Cavagnetto F et al (2012) One-to-one comparison between digital spot compression view and digital breast tomosynthesis. Eur Radiol 22:539–544

Tagliafico A, Mariscotti G, Durando M et al (2015) Characterisation of microcalcification clusters on 2D digital mammography (FFDM) and digital breast tomosynthesis (DBT): does DBT underestimate microcalcification clusters? Results of a multicentre study. Eur Radiol. doi:10.1007/s00330-014-3402-8

Zuley ML, Bandos AI, Ganott MA et al (2013) Digital breast tomosynthesis versus supplemental diagnostic mammographic views for evaluation of noncalcified breast lesions. Radiology 266:89–95

Zuley ML, Guo B, Catullo VJ et al (2014) Comparison of two-dimensional synthesized mammograms versus original digital mammograms alone and in combination with tomosynthesis images. Radiology 271:664–671

# Tomosynthesis and Breast Density

**3**

Alberto Tagliafico and Giulio Tagliafico

## 3.1 What Is Breast Density?

Definition:

- Mammographic breast density is a radiographic representation of the dense fibrous and glandular tissue in the breast relative to fat.

On mammography, the skin of the breast appears radiopaque and, if sufficiently thick, accounts for some portion of tissue density. Breast density is a term strictly related to the radiological appearance of the breast parenchyma and is not related to the physical appearance or firmness of the breast at clinical examination. Figure 3.1 shows the appearance of the breast; normal mature adipocytes are the radiolucent areas seen at mammography, and ducts (epithelium and stroma) are the radiopaque areas on mammography.

In the early 1950s, Leborgne first described different breast density parenchymal patterns that were then classified by Wolfe in 1976. Wolfe raised the hypothesis that different breast parenchymal patterns could have a relation with breast cancer risk. Since then, different classifications have been proposed for breast density: the Tabar classification, Wolfe's parenchymal patterns, and several semiquantitative and quantitative computer-aided methods. The most widely known and adopted classification for a qualitative breast density classification is the BI-RADS lexicon (http://www.acr.org/Quality-Safety/Resources/BIRADS). The Breast Imaging-Reporting and Data

A. Tagliafico, MD (✉)
Department of Experimental Medicine -DIMES, Institute of Anatomy University of Genova, Via de Toni 14, Genoa 16132, Italy
e-mail: alberto.tagliafico@unige.it; albertotagliafico@gmail.com

G. Tagliafico, PhD
Azienda Sanitaria Locale, Genoa, Italy
e-mail: giu.taglia@gmail.com

© Springer International Publishing Switzerland 2016
A. Tagliafico et al. (eds.), *Digital Breast Tomosynthesis: A Practical Approach*,
DOI 10.1007/978-3-319-28631-0_3

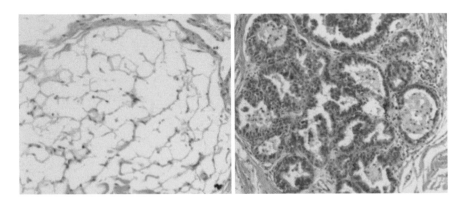

**Fig. 3.1** Photomicrograph (original magnification, 4×; hematoxylin-eosin [H-E] stain) of a breast biopsy specimen shows normal mature adipocytes (*dark areas* seen at mammography) and normal ducts, with ductal epithelium and stromal elements (*white areas* seen at mammography) (Courtesy of Dr. Carli Franca)

System (BI-RADS) classified mammographic density into four categories: the fourth edition of the BI-RADS lexicon created quartiles for each of the four density categories (<25 % glandular, 25–50 % glandular, 51–75 % dense, and >75 % dense, respectively). The quartiles were removed from the BI-RADS fifth edition (http://www.acr.org/Quality-Safety/Resources/BIRADS). To be effective in differentiating women with dense and non-dense breasts, women with "heterogeneously dense" and "extremely dense" are considered "dense," whereas women with "fatty" or "scattered areas of fibroglandular density" are considered "non-dense." According to the last edition of the BI-RADS, the fifth, approximately 50 % of women could be considered as having a dense breast. Therefore, the fifth edition of BI-RADS raised a turf debate as whether it is reasonable to consider so many women at relatively increased risk for developing breast cancer. It is likely that at the time of the release of this book chapter, or in the near future, some adjustments will be made to this statement (Brower 2013; Butler 2015). The importance of breast density received media attention in recent years through the efforts of Nancy Cappello, who was diagnosed with breast cancer without having been informed that she had dense breasts and its implications (Wang et al. 2014). In 2009, Connecticut became the first state to adopt legislation to inform women with dense breast of their relatively increased risk of having a breast cancer. Other states in the United States followed the Connecticut legislation. The increased media attention over breast density has to be accompanied by simple, but crucial, information about a physiological entity that changes over time with ageing:

- Breast density decreases with increasing body mass index (fat content).
- Breast density generally decreases with age.
- Increasing body mass index and ageing increase breast cancer risk.

Other factors such as tamoxifen therapy, hormone replacement therapy, some drugs, weight changes, and dietary changes affect breast density. For this reason, it is possible that a woman has a mammogram reported as dense one year and then non-dense the subsequent year. This situation has to be considered possible due to physiological changes in breast composition. Proper education of the patient and the referring clinician may avoid confusion (Freer 2015).

## 3.2    What Is the Evidence That Breast Density Is a Major Risk Factor for Breast Cancer?

Breast density, considered as mammographic breast density, is a recognized risk factor for breast cancer for two reasons:

- Breast density had a masking effect for breast cancer detection.
- Brest density is an independent risk factor for breast cancer.

### 3.2.1   Masking Effect

A higher number of interval cancers (those diagnosed after a negative mammographic screen and before the next scheduled screen) is thought to be registered in women with dense breast due to the reduced sensitivity of mammography in these patients. Indeed, mammographic sensitivity is reduced from as high as 80–98 % in women with entirely fatty breasts to 30–64.4 % in women with extremely dense breasts (Butler 2015). For this reason, it is suggested that women with dense breasts might benefit from shorter screening intervals and/or through an adjunct imaging modality, usually ultrasound (or potentially tomosynthesis) or even MRI (Emaus et al. 2015).

The sensitivity of screening with mammography plus ultrasound in women with dense breasts was suggested and evaluated in several studies well before the passage of the first breast density legislation in the United States. The ultrasound beam has a physical principle that it is not limited by radiographic density; therefore, ultrasound would be expected to and is capable of detecting cancers that are occult on mammography or tomosynthesis. The masking effect of dense mammographic tissue on breast cancer detection was additionally supported by a recent retrospective review of 335 breast cancers detected at screening US. In this study, it was found that 263/335 cancers (78 %) were missed at mammography probably due to the presence of overlapping dense breast tissue (Bae et al. 2014).

### 3.2.2   Independent Risk Factor for Breast Cancer

Several papers dealing with breast density report that in women with dense breasts, the risk of developing breast cancer is four to six times greater than that of women with dense breasts (Boyd et al. 2007; Yaghjyan et al. 2012; Byrne et al. 1995, 2001; Vachon et al. 2007; McCormack and dos Santos Silva 2006). It is worthy of mention that the risk is very high only when comparing women with extremely dense breasts and at the highest 10 % of density to the lowest 10 % of density being women with almost entirely fatty breasts. When women with heterogeneously dense and extremely dense breasts are compared with women with average breast density, the risk was estimated to be only 1.2–2.1 times greater. Several studies excluded potential confounding factors such as age, menopausal status, hormone use, or therapy and confirmed that breast density is a significant and independent risk factor for breast cancer. A recent study also found an association between increased breast density and higher-grade tumors as well as estrogen receptor-negative tumors (Yaghjyan et al. 2012). A systematic meta-analysis of data for >14,000 cases from 42 studies found that breast density was independently associated with risk of breast cancer (McCormack and dos Santos Silva 2006). Associations were stronger for percentage density rather than for Wolfe categories in the meta-analysis. The breast cancer risk did not differ by age, menopausal status, or ethnicity and cannot be explained by the masking of cancers by dense tissue. Women with the most increased breast density had a risk of breast cancer 4–6 times higher than women with least dense breasts (McCormack and dos Santos Silva 2006). Increased breast density, as evaluated with quantitative methods, is an independent risk factor for breast cancer. Only genetic abnormalities, age, and prior breast cancer are associated with similar or greater relative risk of breast cancer (Harvey and Bovbjerg 2004; McCormack and dos Santos Silva 2006). It is noteworthy that Kavanagh and colleagues (Kavanagh et al. 2008) showed that increasing breast density was associated with risk of breast cancers that have generally poorer prognosis, such as large screen-detected and interval cancers, relative to that of small screen-detected cancers. In this study, the risk of interval cancers increased from the lowest quintile to the highest decile of density, with women in the highest decile estimated to have almost five times the risk of an interval cancer (OR 4.65; 95 % CI 2.96–7.31) relative to those in the lowest quintile. There is also some evidence of a possible association between breast density and breast cancer mortality; however, the association may be limited once adjusted for age, tumor size and grade, node status, and body mass index (Chiu et al. 2010). An open question regarding breast density is if it can be considered a quantitative imaging biomarker. According to the recent report by the RSNA-QIBA Metrology Working Group, a quantitative imaging biomarker is defined as "a characteristic that is objectively measured and evaluated as an indicator of normal biological processes, pathogenic processes, or a response to a therapeutic intervention" (Sullivan et al. 2015). Concordant to this definition, we presume that breast density, if quantitatively assessed, can be included to the list of radiological quantitative imaging biomarkers. The study, validation, and check of imaging biomarkers are gaining importance in the United States and Europe: several scientific societies are devoting resources to this field (European Society of Radiology 2013), and the research field dealing with breast density is particularly active.

## 3.3    How Is Breast Density Best Assessed?

To consider breast density as a quantitative biomarker, the BI-RADS evaluation, which is an ordered scale, is unlikely to be sufficient. Indeed, ordered scales are those for which values are assigned a magnitude and for which there is a meaningful ordering of values; however, neither the difference between any two values nor the ratio of two values is meaningful (Stevens 1946). Breast density assessed using the Breast Imaging-Reporting and Data System, or BI-RADS, for categories 1 (almost entirely fat) through 4 (extremely dense) cannot be considered a quantitative biomarker. The advantages of having breast density assessed as a quantitative biomarker are relevant to the future evolution of precision medicine, which in the United States, has been identified as a national priority (http://www.nih.gov/precisionmedicine/). In precision medicine, biomarker evaluation is crucial for tailoring and monitoring therapy to the individual's molecular signature of the disease. In light of these new horizons, breast density evaluation with continuous and more precise values than the quantitative BI-RADS categories is emerging as a clinical need (Highnam et al. 2007; Diorio et al. 2004). For this reason, it is important to develop a software for quantitative assessment of breast density on standard mammograms, digital mammography, digital breast tomosynthesis, and magnetic resonance imaging. The topic related to breast density and tomosynthesis is relatively new compared to the assessment of breast density on mammography, reflecting the relative novelty of tomosynthesis usage. Indeed, a search for the keywords "breast density and breast cancer" on 18 January 2014 produced 6758 articles, whereas the same search with the keywords "breast density and tomosynthesis" produced only 27 articles. However, the trend in the article published reflects an almost constant and continuous increase of the interest for breast density as shown in Fig. 3.2.

In the recent years, both academic- and industry-related research has developed various softwares to assess breast density quantitatively. Although the purpose of this chapter is not to comprehensively discuss the advantages or disadvantages of any individual software packages, we will list some of the programs that have been applied in this setting and briefly note some of their features; the systems include Quantra, Cumulus, MedDensity, ImageJ, and Volpara. For *Quantra*, one of the first published papers (Ciatto et al. 2012) stated that "Reproducibility was satisfactory on a four (BI-RADS D1-2-3-4) and two grade scale (D1-2 vs. D3-4). Computer-assessed breast density is absolutely reproducible and may be preferred to visual classification. Thus far few studies have addressed the issue of adjusting computer-assessed density to reproduce visual classification, and more similar comparative studies are needed (Ciatto et al. 2012)". However, *Quantra* software provided systematically lower density percentage values as compared to visual classification, and it used only raw data. Cumulus (University of Toronto) and MedDensity (Genova) identify the dense tissue regions on the basis of interactive gray-level thresholding of image pixel values in the following steps: the original image is windowed and leveled interactively, to provide optimal visualization of the dense tissue; then, after pectoral muscle region segmentation, threshold value corresponding to the breast outline is selected interactively. Finally, breast density is

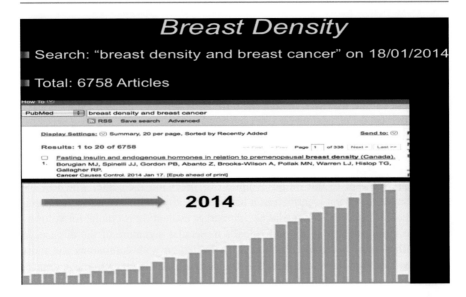

**Fig. 3.2** Trend in the article published on the topic "breast density" which reflects an almost constant and continuous increase of the number of the published articles

given as a percentage. At the time of the present chapter, the relative disadvantages of Cumulus were the absence of capability to analyze 3D images, the absence of a fully automated method to assess breast density, and the influence of breast density percentage results due to variability in breast thickness, variability in breast compression, and variability in X-ray exposure. A notable advantage of the MedDensity software is that it was the first to have an automatic interface to assess also 3D images (of digital breast tomosynthesis) and to assess breast density on magnetic resonance imaging. An example of MedDensity interface is shown in Fig. 3.3. To assess breast density automatically, a recent study found good agreement between an automated software and breast density evaluated by a panel of experts even using a multi-vendor dataset (Sacchetto et al. 2015). A recent review (He et al. 2015) on automatic mammographic density and parenchymal segmentation found that the distribution of various mammographic tissue segmentation approaches from 1992 to 2014 includes 2D projection-based approaches using density for the 80 % of cases, 2D projection-based approaches using parenchymal patterns for 10 % of cases, and, then, the remaining 10 % of cases uses 2D projection-based volumetric approaches or, rarely, 3D reconstruction-based volumetric approaches.

In conclusion, the assessment of breast density involves many issues related to the developed techniques and practicalities that should be faced before bridging translational research to clinical utilization. Various fully automatic mammographic tissue segmentation approaches have been developed or are currently under investigation to overcome subjective estimation of tissue composition, reduce inter- and intra-observer variability, and eliminate ambiguous outcomes (He et al. 2015). In the future, the mammographic tissue segmentation may have a

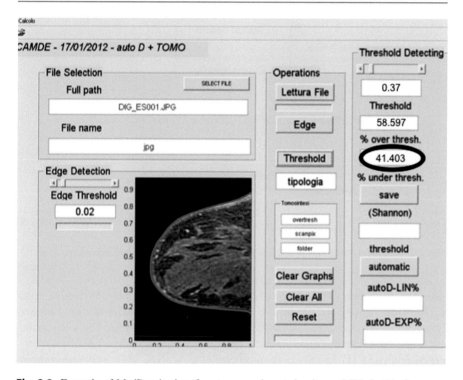

**Fig. 3.3** Example of MedDensity interface to assess breast density on MRI. In this figure, an example of the graphical computer interface is demonstrated. On the left, the edges of the breast are identified (edges are artificially thickened for visual purposes), then the radiologist adjusts the density threshold (semiautomated method) on the right, and finally the percentage of breast density is shown (*black circle*). In this example, the breast result was 41 % dense (From Tagliafico et al. (2014))

strong impact on breast cancer risk prediction. However, nowadays, it has not yet been included in any established risk prediction model (He et al. 2015). The incorporation of quantitative breast density assessment in risk prediction models will be a great step forward to a personalized approach of breast cancer prevention and monitoring.

## 3.4    What Factors Influence Breast Density?

As stated before in Sect. 3.1, it is very important to stress the concept that breast density represents a dynamic physiological entity that changes over time with ageing and under the influence of different substances acting through an endocrine or paracrine mechanisms. The influence of different substances acting as mitogens or mutagens influences breast density and shares some common mechanisms linked with breast cancer development (Fig. 3.4). In normal conditions, breast density decreases with an increasing body mass index (fat content) and breast density

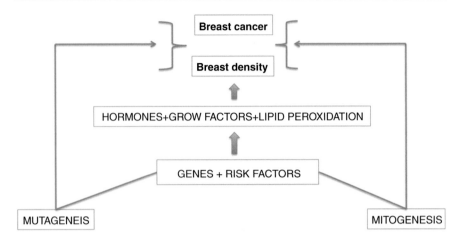

**Fig. 3.4** Scheme showing how breast density could be influenced by mitogens or mutagens

decreases with age. A recent report presented at RSNA 2013 by Perry et al. compared breast density and cancer risk between younger and older women and analyzed how the risk relates to changes in breast density over time. The study group evaluated breast density quantitatively on digital mammography in 282 breast cancer patients and 317 healthy controls (Perry et al. RSNA, 2013, personal communication). It was found that patients affected by breast cancer had higher mammographic density than healthy participants up to the age of 50. Then, the healthy controls showed a decline in density with age with a linear pattern, as normally happens with ageing, whereas there was considerably more variability in density regression among the breast cancer patients who often did not show a decrease in breast density. According to Perry's work, different biological density mechanisms for normal breasts compared to breasts with cancer could be hypothesized. This study, along with other studies reporting several factors influencing breast density (growth hormone, insulin-like growth factors, binding proteins, drugs such as tamoxifen), suggests that breast density is indeed a unique and important risk factor for breast cancer. Indeed, a recent meta-analysis of five genome-wide association studies (GWAS) identified variants within the intron 4 of the ZNF365 gene that are associated with both high breast density and higher breast cancer risk (Lindstrom et al. 2011). A new study by (Stone et al. 2015) suggested that 18 % of breast cancer susceptibility genomic variants for breast cancer were associated with at least one mammographic density measure. Genetic variants at multiple loci were associated with both breast cancer risk and mammographic density measures. This study used data for 10,727 women and estimated associations between 77 common breast cancer susceptibility variants and absolute dense area, percent dense area, and absolute non-dense area. The data were adjusted for age and body mass index.

## 3.5    How Do You Utilize Breast Density in the Preventive Setting?

At the time of the present chapter, there are no formal guidelines or recommendations on how to use breast density in preventive medicine. Indeed, the legislations approved in the United States, requiring that women with increased breast density have to be informed about their risk of developing or having breast cancer, do not indicate how to use breast density in the preventive setting. Scientific societies, both European and American, are starting to consider breast density as an important biomarker, especially if measured quantitatively. The topic related to the use of breast density as a quantitative biomarker is rapidly expanding in the medical literature as shown in Fig. 3.2, and there are some topics in which quantitative assessment of breast can be considered promising. In this paragraph, we simply list some of the research topics appearing in the literature that seem most relevant for clinical practice (Diorio et al. 2004; Highnam et al. 2007):

- Epidemiological studies including the estimation of breast cancer risk
- Radiation dose monitoring
- Effects of hormone replacement therapy (HRT)
- Effects of different hormones (GH/FSH/IGF-I, etc.)
- Effects of growth factors (IGF-I/IGF-I BP, etc.)
- Chemoprevention (TAM low dose, 5 mg vs. 25 mg: Trial of Low Dose Tamoxifen in Women With Breast Intraepithelial Neoplasia (TAM-01); NCT01357772)

Here we review one example from the prevention studies related to breast density and that uses tamoxifen as chemoprevention (Cuzick et al. 2011): the International Breast Cancer Intervention Study I (IBIS I) has reported that for women on tamoxifen who had a reduction in breast density of 10 % or more, breast cancer risk was significantly reduced by 52 % relative to controls. Women on tamoxifen who had a reduction in breast density of less than 10 % had a small reduction in breast cancer incidence to be confirmed by further evidence. A measurable change in mammographic density at 12- to 18-month appears to be a good predictor of response to tamoxifen in the preventive setting. The IBIS I example is only one possible demonstration of how breast density can be used in a clinical setting to guide and monitor different therapies. Another example is the demonstration of increased breast density in acromegalic patients (Tagliafico et al. 2011). In these patients, mammographic breast density in premenopausal patients was significantly higher than controls and positively correlated with IGF-I and disease duration. For this reason, we suggest that, according to the principle that when mammographic density is included in clinical risk models, more women may be eligible for supplemental screening methods (such as screening MRI and WB-US) because including density in such risk models may improve the ability to identify those at increased risk. We anticipate that the amount of information on how to use breast density in a preventive clinical setting will expand considerably in future years.

## 3.6    Measurement of Breast Density with Digital Breast Tomosynthesis

Digital breast tomosynthesis (DBT) is rapidly being implemented in the screening and diagnostic settings for breast cancer. The number of clinical trials supporting the role of DBT in clinical practice is growing fast (see Chaps. 2 and 4), although some studies report its limitations in assessing microcalcification (Tagliafico A, Houssami N et al. 2015 and Chapter 2). DBT was approved by the US Food and Drug Administration in 2011. Large-scale studies of screening DBT in the real-world clinical setting have repeatedly shown an increase in cancer detection and a significant reduction in recall rates compared with the use of traditional two-dimensional digital mammography at first (prevalent) screening examination, likely as a direct result of a decreased masking effect. The decrease in masking effect is a surrogate of a reduction in breast density as assessed by DBT. Indeed, DBT uses a series of low-dose mammograms acquired over an arc to reconstruct the breast in thin tissue planes that reduce the superimposition of overlapping radiopaque dense/fibroglandular breast tissue. For this reason, it is not surprising that one of the first studies comparing breast density assessed on MMX and DBT reported lower values for breast density measurement compared to 2D (Tagliafico et al. 2012). In this study, which is limited by the fact that most patients had dense breasts (meaning that the study series did not have the normal distribution in the classical BI-RADS density categories), the values of breast density were lower on DBT than those obtained on standard mammography (Fig. 3.5). A recent study tried to fill the gap in knowledge on how breast density estimation might differ between MMX and DBT across all BI-RADS density categories (Tagliafico et al. 2013a, b). This study was a prospective study of diagnostic women who underwent both DBT and MMX. Forty patients in each BI-RADS category were enrolled, and the categories were determined according a classical BI-RADS distribution based on the fourth edition (D1: 0–25 %, D2: 26–50 %, D3:51–75 % and D4:>76 %). This study found that using DBT, breast density values were significantly lower than those obtained using MMx ($p < 0.0001$), with a nonlinear relationship across the BI-RADS categories as shown in Fig. 3.6. Relative to DBT:

- In BI-RADS class 1, digital mammography overestimated BD by 16 %.
- In BI-RADS class 2, digital mammography overestimated BD by 11.9 %.
- In BI-RADS class 3, digital mammography overestimated BD by 3.5 %.
- In BI-RADS class 4, digital mammography overestimated BD by 18.1 %.

These data have to be considered in clinical practice and research studies using breast density as a possible biomarker in determining the risk of developing breast cancer. Indeed, it is possible that a woman with dense breasts has a difference in breast density percentage assessed with software of up to 18 % due to the different mammographic techniques, DBT or MMx, adopted to estimate breast density. In a clinical study assessing breast density that might cross modalities in measuring breast density over time or in different patients, knowledge of these differences are

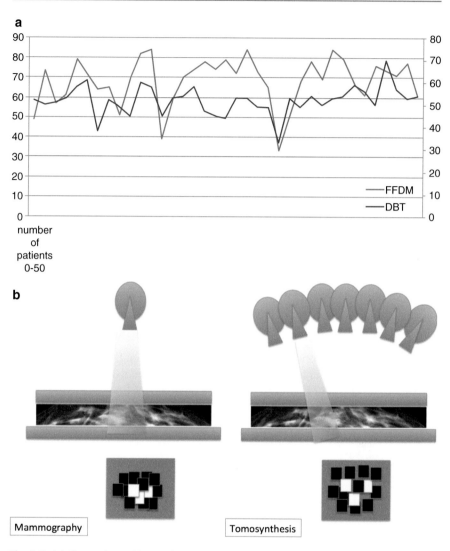

**Fig. 3.5** (**a**) Comparison of breast density values estimated with the maximum entropy method (*FFDM* full-field digital mammography, *DBT* digital breast tomosynthesis). As shown by the graph, breast density appeared to be significantly underestimated on digital breast tomosynthesis (*purple line*) (From: Tagliafico et al. (2012), with permission). In (**b**) the scheme should help to understand how breast density could be underestimated on DBT compared to FFDM

useful to correct discrepancies not due to physiological phenomena but resulting from the technique used. There are different methods to assess breast density on DBT. All of these methods have been used in different clinical or research studies with different purposes: to assess diagnostic performance of DBT and MMx in different classes of breast density or to compare breast density in patients who had both DBT and MMx. At the time of the present chapter, we are not aware of any

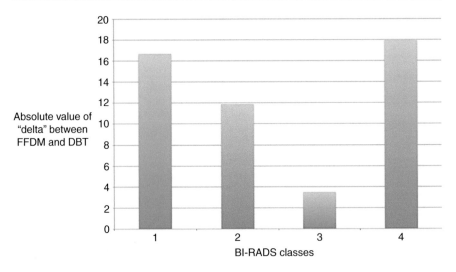

**Fig. 3.6** Differences in the delta between two-dimensional full-field digital mammography (2D *FFDM*) and digital breast tomosynthesis (*DBT*) according to Breast Imaging-Reporting and Data System (*BI-RADS*) categories. The y-axis shows the percentage density (From Tagliafico et al. (2013a), with permission)

relevant clinical study correlating breast density assessed on DBT with breast cancer risk. Indeed, at present, we do not know if breast cancer risk is more accurately assessed using DBT or MMX, and this would be worthy of future research.

The methods used to assess breast density on DBT are:

- Qualitative using a classical BI-RADS scale
- Semiquantitative with software
- Quantitative with automated software

Each method has advantages and disadvantages. A recent systematic review dealing with measurement of breast density with digital breast tomosynthesis (Ekpo and McEntee 2014) confirmed that the poor reproducibility of the BI-RADS system applied to breast density evaluation on DBT may have implications on breast cancer risk prediction and choices in screening. Objective measurements of breast density with quantitative approaches developed for breast density evaluation include semi-automated and fully automated methods.

Semiautomated methods mainly use thresholding and segmentation techniques such as Cumulus, MedDensity, and Madena. These methods assess the borders of the breast and mammographic percentage density using an interface where the reader or the radiologist can adjust the threshold to best differentiate fat from parenchyma or dense from non-dense tissue. Of the available semiautomated methods, only Cumulus and MedDensity have been used for breast density estimation with DBT. Computerized thresholding and segmentation techniques select gray levels for density assessment from the central DBT image slice (Cumulus) or from every slice (MedDensity). Usually, two gray levels are usually selected to separate the fibroglandular (dense) breast tissue from the non-dense background. The software then calculates percentage breast density as the percentage of the dense tissue and the total breast area. The software worked with good intra- and inter-observer agreement. According to the recent review by Ekpo et al., the softwares used most frequently were Autodensity, MedDensity (the automated version), SMF, Volpara, and Quantra. MedDensity gave an area measurement of breast density as percentages; Volpara and Quantra measured volumetric breast density and graded such densities into BI-RADS categories. MedDensity (developed by Giulio Tagliafico, University of Genova, Italy) is a method based on maximum entropy and uses the spatial information for automatic thresholding and segmentation of breast into fatty and dense tissue. It calculates percentage breast density as the percentage of the area of the dense tissue or non-dense tissue. MedDensity has shown breast density evaluated with DBT to be lower than that for DM by 11.4 % and the level of breast density underestimation with DBT varying according to BI-RADS categories: 16.0 %, 11.0 %, 3.5 %, and 18.1 % for BI-RADS 1, 2, 3, and 4, respectively. MedDensity has an automated interface, but noise in the image limits the thresholding capability and can reduce the reliability of the software. Volpara (Volpara Solutions, Mātakina Company, Wellington, New Zealand) estimates breast density by finding a reference point of entirely fat in each image and then estimating X-ray attenuation relative to that point for all other points in the image. Then, the software calculates the volume of dense tissue by integrating the thickness of the dense tissue at each pixel level values over the image. Volpara calculates average percentage volumetric breast density as a percentage of the volume of fibroglandular tissue and the total volume of the breast. It seems that Volpara also generates relatively lower density values than BI-RADS. Quantra (Hologic Inc., Bedford, MA), to the best of our present knowledge, has not been used for breast density estimation with DBT so far. In conclusion, although several issues regarding breast density on DBT are still to be clarified, it could be suggested that an automated, reader-friendly, and standardized breast density measurement could be easily introduced in both research and clinical settings.

## 3.7 Breast Density Assessment Using Mammography, Tomosynthesis, and MRI and Their Implications for Practice

The majority of knowledge about breast tissue density derives from conventional mammography.

Studies comparing mammographic breast density measurements with those obtained on DBT or MRI are few and generally highlight some differences among the three techniques. However, having knowledge of how these modalities can be used to compare breast density values is important where the screening of breast cancer is personalized and starts at an early age with non-X-ray techniques such as MRI (e.g., high-risk females). The future of research on this topic should establish how to compare measurement of breast density on different modalities used in clinical practice, including ultrasound that is often used in young women. Also, today, it is not known which modality best predicts the risk of breast cancer through measuring breast density. As an example of what can be done in a research setting, a recent study assessed breast density by means of DBT, MMx, and MRI on the same patient (Tagliafico et al. 2013a, b). This study found that:

- *MMX overestimated breast density in 15.1% in comparison to DBT and in 16.2% in comparison to MRI.*
- The *mean values* and standard deviation of percentage breast density were 66.1 ± 22.2 for MMx, 54.3 ± 21.5 for DBT, and 53.4 ± 21.5.
- Differences in breast percentage between *MRI and DBT* were found to be *not statistically significant* ($p > 0.05$).

Therefore, breast density evaluated on DBT may be considered similar to the results obtained by MRI (Fig. 3.7) which could be one of the best reference standards available considering that, for practical reasons, a true histological reference standard is not achievable. We also tried to suggest a way to compare breast density among different modalities by using formulas. For example, MRI percent density = 0.3198 + 0.9848 DBT percent density (Tagliafico et al. 2013a, b). However, this formula is far from being validated, and it has to be considered only for demonstrative purposes, and further work has to be done to find the best way to compare breast density across different modalities.

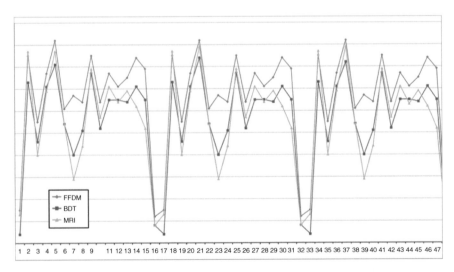

**Fig. 3.7** Comparison of breast density values (percent) estimated with maximum entropy thresholding method for three breast imaging modalities (*FFDM* full-field digital mammography, *DBT* digital breast Tomosynthesis, *MRI* magnetic resonance imaging) (Reprinted with permission from: Tagliafico et al. (2013b))

# References

Bae MS, Moon WK, Chang JM et al (2014) Breast cancer detected with screening US: reasons for nondetection at mammography. Radiology 270:369–377

Boyd NF, Guo H, Martin LJ et al (2007) Mammographic density and the risk and detection of breast cancer. N Engl J Med 356:227–236

Brower V (2013) Breast density legislation fueling controversy. J Natl Cancer Inst 105:510–511

Butler RS (2015) Invited commentary: the breast density dilemma – challenges, lessons, and future directions. Radiographics 35:324–326

Byrne C, Schairer C, Wolfe J et al (1995) Mammographic features and breast cancer risk: effects with time, age, and menopause status. J Natl Cancer Inst 87:1622–1629

Byrne C, Schairer C, Brinton LA et al (2001) Effects of mammographic density and benign breast disease on breast cancer risk (United States). Cancer Causes Control 12(2):103–110

Chiu SYH, Duffy S, Yen AMF, Tabar L, Smith RA, Chen HH (2010) Effect of baseline breast density on breast cancer incidence, stage, mortality, and screening parameters: 25-Year follow-up of a Swedish mammographic screening. Cancer Epidemiol Biomarkers Prev 19(5):1219–1228

Ciatto S, Bernardi D, Calabrese M et al (2012) A first evaluation of breast radiological density assessment by QUANTRA software as compared to visual classification. Breast 21:503–506

Cuzick J, Warwick J, Pinney E et al (2011) Tamoxifen-induced reduction in mammographic density and breast cancer risk reduction: a Nested Case–Control Study. J Natl Cancer Inst 103:744–752

Diorio C, Pollak M, Byrne C et al (2004) Insulin-like growth factor-I, IGF-binding protein-3, and mammographic breast density. Cancer Epidemiol Biomarkers Prev 14:1065–1073

Ekpo EU, McEntee MF (2014) Measurement of breast density with digital breast tomosynthesis – a systematic review. Br J Radiol 87(1043):20140460

Emaus MJ, Bakker MF, Peeters PH et al (2015) MR imaging as an additional screening modality for the detection of breast cancer in women aged 50–75 years with extremely dense breasts: the DENSE trial study design. Radiology. 277(2):527–37. doi: 10.1148/radiol.2015141827

European Society of Radiology (ESR) (2013) ESR statement on the stepwise development of imaging biomarkers. Insights Imaging 4:147–152

Freer PE (2015) Mammographic breast density: impact on breast cancer risk and implications for screening. Radiographics 35:302–315

Harvey JA, Bovbjerg VE (2004) Quantitative assessment of mammographic breast density: relationship with breast cancer risk. Radiology 230:29–41

He W, Juette A, Denton ER et al (2015) A review on automatic mammographic density and parenchymal segmentation. Int J Breast Cancer 2015:276217. doi:10.1155/2015/276217, Epub 2015 Jun 11

Highnam R, Jeffreys M, McCormack V et al (2007) Comparing measurements of breast density. Phys Med Biol 52:5881–5895

Kavanagh AM, Byrnes GB, Nickson C et al (2008) Using mammographic density to improve breast cancer screening outcomes. Cancer Epidemiol Biomarkers Prev 17(10):2818–2824

Lindstrom S, Vachon CM, Li J et al (2011) Common variants in ZNF365 are associated with both mammographic density and breast cancer risk. Nat Genet 43:185–187

McCormack VA, dos Santos Silva I (2006) Breast density and parenchymal patterns as markers of breast cancer risk: a meta-analysis. Cancer Epidemiol Biomarkers Prev 15:1159–1169

Sacchetto D, Morra L, Agliozzo S et al (2015) Mammographic density: comparison of visual assessment with fully automatic calculation on a multivendor dataset. Eur Radiol. 26(1):175–83. doi: 10.1007/s00330-015-3784-2

Stevens SS (1946) On the theory of scales of measurement. Science 103:677–680

Stone J, Thompson DJ, Dos Santos Silva I et al (2015) Novel associations between common breast cancer susceptibility variants and risk-predicting mammographic density measures. Cancer Res 75:2457–2467

Sullivan DC, Obuchowski NA, Kessler LG, et al, RSNA-QIBA Metrology Working Group. (2015) Metrology standards for quantitative imaging biomarkers. Radiology. 277(3):813–25. doi: 10.1148/radiol.2015142202

Tagliafico A, Houssami N (2015) Digital breast tomosynthesis might not be the optimal modality for detecting microcalcification. Radiology 275:618–619

Tagliafico A, Calabrese M, Tagliafico G et al (2011) Increased mammographic breast density in acromegaly: quantitative and qualitative assessment. Eur J Endocrinol 164:335–340

Tagliafico A, Tagliafico G, Astengo D et al (2012) Mammographic density estimation: one-to-one comparison of digital mammography and digital breast tomosynthesis using fully automated software. Eur Radiol 22:1265–1270

Tagliafico AS, Tagliafico G, Cavagnetto F et al (2013a) Estimation of percentage breast tissue density: comparison between digital mammography (2D full field digital mammography) and digital breast tomosynthesis according to different BI-RADS categories. Br J Radiol 86(1031):20130255

Tagliafico A, Tagliafico G, Astengo D et al (2013b) Comparative estimation of percentage breast tissue density for digital mammography, digital breast tomosynthesis, and magnetic resonance imaging. Breast Cancer Res Treat 138:311–317. doi:10.1007/s10549-013-2419-z

Tagliafico A et al (2014) Breast density assessment using a 3T MRI system: comparison among different sequences. PLoS One 9(6):e99027

Tagliafico A, Mariscotti G, Durando M et al (2015) Characterisation of microcalcification clusters on 2D digital mammography (FFDM) and digital breast tomosynthesis (DBT): does DBT underestimate microcalcification clusters? Results of a multicentre study. Eur Radiol 25:9–14

Vachon CM, van Gils CH, Sellers TA et al (2007) Mammographic density, breast cancer risk and risk prediction. Breast Cancer Res 9:217

Wang AT, Vachon CM, Brandt KR, Ghosh K (2014) Breast density and breast cancer risk: a practical review. Mayo Clin Proc 89:548–557

Yaghjyan L, Colditz GA, Rosner B, Tamimi RM (2012) Mammographic breast density and breast cancer risk by menopausal status, postmenopausal hormone use and a family history of breast cancer. Cancer Causes Control 23:785–790

# Clinical Applications for Digital Breast Tomosynthesis

# 4

Luca A. Carbonaro

## 4.1 Introduction

The use of digital breast tomosynthesis (DBT) associated to digital mammography (DM) in screening has been proved to increase the detection rate and to reduce recall rates (Skaane et al. 2013; Ciatto et al. 2013) although the effect on recall rates varies according to the recall rules (Ciatto et al. 2013). See also Chap. 2 by Per Skaane for applications of DBT in screening.

DBT is a relatively new and still evolving technique, and DBT systems are still not widely available nor widely implemented, and few systems in practice have the capability to generate a synthetic 2D reconstructed mammogram from 3D tomosynthetic images.

At present, there are no consensus guidelines about practical use of DBT imaging and no clear indications on which population could benefit the best from it; however, evidence on DBT in use other than screening indicates that DBT images may help the radiologist in some applications:

- The workup of patients with a suspicious finding at (screen film or digital) mammography
- The local staging of a newly diagnosed breast cancer
- The "second-look" evaluation of a suspicious finding at breast magnetic resonance imaging

However, while the evidence on the use of DBT in clinical applications (other than screening) will be outlined in this chapter, it should be noted that the evidence is still generally limited to a few studies and that many studies are cancer enriched

L.A. Carbonaro, MD
Radiology Unit, IRCCS Policlinico San Donato,
Via Morandi 30, San Donato Milanese (MI) 20097, Italy
e-mail: luca.carbonaro@gmail.com

© Springer International Publishing Switzerland 2016
A. Tagliafico et al. (eds.), *Digital Breast Tomosynthesis: A Practical Approach*,
DOI 10.1007/978-3-319-28631-0_4

and/or conducted retrospectively, which means there is some risk that reported results are affected by bias.

## 4.2    Digital Breast Tomosynthesis in Clinical Workup of Suspicious Mammographic Findings

Reading a mammogram can be considered a two-step process, which consists in detection and diagnostic evaluation of any abnormal finding on the image. After a finding on mammography has been detected and described as suspicious, the traditional workup is usually composed by additional mammographic views followed by a targeted breast ultrasonography (US), if needed (Harvey et al. 2008).

The use of a mammographic view with spot compression can better evaluate abnormalities such as microcalcifications, masses, or architectural distortions and to distinguish true from fictitious findings (false positives at screening) created by superimposed areas of normal breast tissue (Sickles 1989). The use of DBT permits cross-sectional visualization of breast tissue, reducing the difficulty caused by the superimposition or overlapping of tissue (Gur et al. 2009). By consequence, lesions have a better conspicuity at DBT images, and the use of tomosynthesis has been proved to have a diagnostic accuracy at least equal to that of digital spot compression in three studies (Noroozian et al. 2012; Tagliafico et al. 2012; Zuley et al. 2013). The use of DBT images allowed the radiologist to decrease the number of lesions classified as BI-RADS category 3, particularly masses and asymmetries, with a concomitant substantial increase in the number of lesions categorized as BI-RADS 1, BI-RADS 2, or BI-RADS 5 (Zuley et al. 2013). In clinical practice, the use of tomosynthesis is likely to translate into fewer short interval follow-up studies and may possibly lead to fewer biopsies in patients with benign lesions. The technical execution of spot compression views is not always perfect due to problems in aiming the mammographic finding, especially in large breasts, which can result in the repetition of spot views, with consequent higher patient's distress along with higher radiation exposure, or worst in a diagnostic error for an unnoticed lesion outside the spot compression image. On the contrary, a DBT exam shows simultaneously the whole breast, without the need of a specific target; this approach erases this technical difficulty of positioning the patient and results in a very good intra- and interobserver agreement for the radiologists (Tagliafico et al. 2012). Furthermore, in cases where more than one finding is detected in different breast quadrants, DBT obviates the need to repeat a spot compression view for every lesion.

Tomosynthesis has been studied for any type of mammographic finding, and BI-RADS lexicon for mammography (D'Orsi et al. 2013) can be applied easily to DBT images. This technique showed a better sensitivity than spot compression imaging (about 94 % versus 50.2 %) in focal asymmetries for lesion visualization and differentiation of true lesions from summation artifacts (ElMaadawy et al. 2012). Some advantages can be found in the evaluation of architectural distortion with DBT, which allows the radiologist to better visualize the radiating lines that converge to a point, and it is especially useful in discriminating a possible distortion along a fat-glandular interface from anatomical fibrotic tissue (Peppard et al. 2015). When a mass has been detected in mammography, it might be characterized by shape, margin, and density. Shape and margins of benign and malignant masses appear better defined at DBT, which allows a reclassification of the degree of suspicion with a lower BI-RADS category for benign lesions and a higher BI-RADS category for malignant lesions (Zuley et al. 2013). Brandt and colleagues suggested that DBT can replace additional mammographic views for the evaluation of noncalcified findings recalled from screening mammography with similar sensitivity and specificity for the two techniques (Brandt et al. 2013). On the other hand, tomosynthesis might have a more limited role in the workup of microcalcifications, as the data are not established regarding the detectability of this finding with DBT, where the sensitivity of DBT has been shown to be somewhat inferior to that of DM (Spangler et al. 2011; Kopans et al. 2011; Tagliafico et al. 2015). In fact, it could be difficult to identify a group of microcalcification with DBT images alone when only few microcalcifications are laying on the same DBT slice. Nonetheless, the 3D evaluation performed by DBT, obtained by scrolling through the image slices, may help the radiologist to better define the distribution and the distance between more clusters of microcalcifications. Tomosynthesis, as well as zoomed images from DM, cannot serve as an alternative to direct mammographic magnification view, which proved to show a better definition of microcalcification shape and morphology (Kim et al. 2009).

The 3D evaluation in DBT appears to be particularly helpful when a finding is best imaged on one view only (or not seen at all, as in the axillary tail of mediolateral oblique views, as in the inner quadrants of craniocaudal views): the radiologist can find the lesion's position in relation of the slice number where the abnormality is best visualized, with lower numbers being inferior on the craniocaudal view and lateral on the mediolateral view. The use of DBT images appears to be a potential replacement of the conventional "rolled" mammographic views, in which the breast is rolled either medial or lateral in the CC projection and the subsequent direction in which the lesion moves on each rolled CC view provides a clue to the true lesion location (Harvey et al. 2008). Knowing where to look helps to identify and further characterize the lesion, including using this information to guide the US examination to the correct anatomic location in the breast for subsequent sonographic characterization and ultrasound-guided biopsy (Cohen 2014).

Tomosynthesis is a technique based on the same physical principles of DM yet with better specificity than mammography alone (Zuley et al. 2013), due to its capability to better define shape and margins of most lesions; DBT however is not sufficient to evaluate a mass density with the same capability as US. In the clinical setting, the role of US is complementary to both DM and DBT because it can offer additional information about the features of a lesion (such as solid-cystic differentiation or suspicious signs). Moreover, US can detect additional cancers unseen on conventional DM, particularly at age <50 years, in women with previous breast cancer and in dense breasts (i.e., with ACR density patterns C and D (D'Orsi et al. 2013); (Girardi et al. 2013)). In a retrospective study of an enriched sample of 1042 patients, Elizalde and colleagues proved that diagnostic accuracy of DM was equally improved by adjunct of US or DBT ($p=0.7$) (Elizalde et al. 2014). The authors also showed a further gain in sensitivity (up to almost 99 % versus less than 93 %) when all the three techniques (DM, DBT, and US) have been used in combination. The synergic use of both DBT and US has been proved to obtain a higher sensitivity (75 % versus 50–52 %) also when applied as "second look" after a breast MRI examination, compared to DBT or US techniques alone (Clauser et al. 2015). The reason of this "added" sensitivity is due to the intrinsic technical differences between DBT and US, which can allow radiologists to detect an amount of lesions which show features visible just at one of these techniques and unnoticed (or misdiagnosed) at the other (Kim et al. 2015).

First results have been expected from a non-randomized study, "Tomosynthesis Versus Ultrasonography in Women With Dense Breast (ASTOUND)," whose aim is to demonstrate at least equivalence, or nonsignificant difference between DBT and US in women with dense breast screened negative at 2D mammography. The leader center is the University of Genoa, Italy, in collaboration with the University of Sydney, Australia, and if the equivalence between DBT and US will be demonstrated, US may be substituted by DBT with great benefits for the patients and for the healthcare resources. Information about this study can be retrieved at https://clinicaltrials.gov/ct2/show/study/NCT02066142?term=ASTOUND&rank=1&view=record.

- *In clinical workup, digital breast tomosynthesis is comparable to additional mammographic views in terms of diagnostic accuracy in the evaluation of mammographic findings such as architectural distortions, focal asymmetries, and masses.*
- *Data regarding the detectability of microcalcifications with digital breast tomosynthesis are not established, considering the fundamental role of direct magnification mammography in the evaluation of microcalcifications' shape and distribution.*
- *Digital breast tomosynthesis is complementary (and not alternative) to ultrasound examination.*

## 4.3    Digital Breast Tomosynthesis in Local Staging and Preoperative Setting

The aim of breast imaging is not only to identify breast cancers but to guide their therapy, could it be surgical (and radiotherapeutic) or chemotherapeutic. A correct preoperative evaluation of breast cancer lesions could help the surgeon in the surgical planning showing the site and the extension of the disease and providing information on possible multifocality or multicentricity. In presurgical setting, breast MRI has proved to be the technique of choice, due to the highest sensitivity compared with mammography and ultrasound (Houssami et al. 2008). Nonetheless, present guidelines (ACR Guidelines and Standards Committee et al. 2008; Mann et al. 2008a, b; Sardanelli et al. 2010) recommend the use of breast MRI for local staging only for specific types of breast cancers such as invasive lobular cancers or in specific indications such as for women who are at higher risk of breast cancer or women younger than 60 years old with discrepancy in tumor size >1 cm between mammography and ultrasonography.

Considering that invasive lobular cancers and breast cancers affecting high-risk women are, respectively, about 5–15 % (Orvieto et al. 2008) and 3–5 % (Sardanelli et al. 2010) of all breast cancers and that breast cancer incidence is higher in older population (Althuis et al. 2005), a large quote of women with newly diagnosed breast cancer does not show indication to perform a breast MRI. Furthermore, fast and convenient access to breast MRI is not often available; also more frequent use of preoperative MRI could lead to unnecessary radical surgery for some women (Houssami et al. 2008). Hence clinical breast examination, mammography, and US are the only techniques used for the preoperative evaluation of the majority of breast cancer patients.

In this context, how could digital breast tomosynthesis be helpful in the presurgical local staging?

First of all, the task of the radiologist is to assess the size of the lesion, which is sometimes difficult to evaluate in mammography, especially when overimposed breast tissue can obscure the lesion's margins. The possibility to evaluate individual sections of the breast tissue showed by DBT allows the radiologist to remove overlying and underlying anatomical tissue and, by consequence, to depict more clearly the lesion's margins (Niklason et al. 1997). The result is a better cancer visibility on digital breast tomosynthesis than on DM, as reported by Andersson and colleagues (2008), and consequently a superiority of DBT for the evaluation of the lesion size, as showed by Förnvik and colleagues in a comparison between DBT, DM, and US (Förnvik et al. 2010). They studied 73 diagnosed breast cancers for which the longest diameter at pathology was used as reference standard. The tumor outline could be determined in significantly more cases with DBT ($n=63$) and ultrasound ($n=60$) than DM ($n=49$). Digital breast tomosynthesis and US size correlated well with pathology ($R=0.86$ and $R=0.85$, respectively) and significantly better than mammographic size ($R=0.71$). The cancer size underestimation of all the imaging techniques used was mainly due to the conservative approximation of the tumor outline used by the authors, for the impossibility to determine how much of a spicule was tumor growth and how much was reactive fibrosis. On the contrary, the authors noted an overestimation of tumor size in the presence of extensive DCIS component, which is well recognizable and precisely measurable at mammography and tomosynthesis in the correspondence of microcalcifications, but barely measurable on pathology, due to their small size and often scattered distribution (Förnvik et al. 2010).

In a later and larger study, Mun and colleagues evaluated 173 malignant breast lesions (with a mean size 23.8 mm, 43 % of them ≤2 cm in size) in 169 patients, which were measured by three radiologists on craniocaudal and mediolateral oblique views of DM and on mediolateral oblique view of tomosynthesis (Mun et al. 2013). The longest diameter measured in the mammographic images and in tomosynthetic images for each lesion was compared to the corresponding longest diameter at pathological examination, and a mis-sized was considered when a difference greater than 1 cm would be found. Overall, the percentage of lesions mis-sized at DBT was significantly lower than at DM (19 % versus 29 %, $p=0.003$). Digital breast tomosynthesis also had significantly less mis-sizing than FFDM in the subgroup of lesions that were less then 2 cm in size (14.7 % difference, $p=0.005$), but no significant mis-sizing difference was found for lesions larger than 2 cm in size ($p=0.153$). The population studied by Mun and colleagues showed that mainly heterogeneously dense breasts (81/173, 47 %) or extremely dense breast (38/173, 22 %) parenchyma and fatty breasts (18/173, 10 %) or scattered fibroglandular breasts (36/173, 21 %) were less common. The authors found that there was consistently less mis-sizing by DBT versus DM across all breast densities, but the difference was not significant for fatty or scattered fibroglandular breasts, while it was in both heterogeneously dense breasts (11.1 % difference between DBT and FFDM, $p$ ¼$=0.016$) and extremely dense breasts (15.8 % difference, $p=0.024$) (Mun et al. 2013). This result confirms the advantage of DBT in overcoming the glandular superimposition that usually affects mammography, which is mostly in heterogeneously and extremely dense breasts. Nonetheless, DBT might have a higher accuracy of lesion's size measurement than mammography even in fatty or scattered fibroglandular breasts, as confirmed by Luparia and colleagues (2013), and the not significant differences between the two techniques could have been the result of the small subgroup population studied by Mun and colleagues (2013).

A comparison between DBT, DM, US, and breast MRI was performed by Luparia and colleagues (2013). They retrospectively evaluated 149 breast cancers in 110 women, comparing the longest diameter at imaging with the pathological report; the measurements were considered concordant if they were within ±5 mm. The Pearson's correlation coefficient of DBT and breast MRI measurements had a better correlation with pathological tumor size ($R=0.89$ and $R=0.92$, respectively) compared to DM ($R=0.83$) and US ($R=0.77$), without any statistical differences between the correlation of DBT and breast MRI. Notably, the authors proved that the correlation coefficient of DM added to DBT ($R=0.89$) was the same as the correlation coefficient of DBT alone ($R=0.89$); this result suggests that measures with DBT were determinant. As for mammographic density, patients were divided into two groups: fatty breasts (ACR 1+ACR 2) and dense breasts (ACR 3+ACR 4). Even if Pearson's correlation coefficients between the lesion measurements performed by DM, DBT, US, and MRI compared to pathological size of the breasts were higher for fatty breasts (0.87, 0.9, 0.83, and 0.94, respectively) than for dense breasts (0.78, 0.87, 0.74, and 0.89, respectively), the difference between the two subgroups was not statistically significant for any modality ($p>0.01$). It confirmed the advantages in using DBT in lesion's measurement not only in dense breasts but in fatty breasts also. Considering different types of cancers, the authors showed a better Pearson's correlation coefficient for DBT than for DM not only for invasive ductal cancers ($R=0.86$ and $R=0.76$, respectively) but also for invasive lobular cancers ($R=0.91$ and $R=0.80$, respectively), without any statistical differences from Pearson's correlation coefficient for MRI colleagues (Luparia et al. 2013). This makes DBT comparable to MRI for preoperative staging for this specific type of tumor, for which MRI proved to be the most effective imaging technique (Mann et al. 2008a, b; Sardanelli et al. 2010). By contrast, DM had a much lower coefficient ($R=0.80$) probably due to the particular presentation of invasive lobular cancer, which is often associated with the presence of parenchymal distortion at mammography; for this reason, it is more difficult to assess the real extent of the tumor margins. As already reported by Mun and colleagues (2013), a higher correlation coefficient with pathological measurements was found for smaller lesions (T1) than for larger lesions (T2) for all the imaging techniques.

Luparia and colleagues also evaluated the detection rate of DM, DBT, US, and MRI in multifocal breast cancers (70 %, 78 %, 75 %, and 94 %, respectively), showing the better performance of breast MRI in the diagnosis of nonunifocal disease (statistically significant, $p<0.01$) (Luparia et al. 2013), as already reported in the literature (Houssami et al. 2008). Digital breast tomosynthesis showed a higher detection rate than DM and US, but these differences were statistically significant ($p>0.01$). These results were confirmed by another study from the same group, in which Mariscotti and colleagues evaluated the accuracy of mammography, DBT, US and MRI in preoperative assessment of 200 consecutive women, prospectively enrolled with newly diagnosed breast cancer (Mariscotti et al. 2014). As previously reported, the authors showed a slightly higher sensitivity and accuracy of DBT (91 % and 90 %, respectively) than DM alone (85 % and 87 %, respectively) for breast cancer staging, but without any significant differences ($p>0.05$). Furthermore, they confirmed that both DM and DBT alone have a lower diagnostic performance than breast MRI. Anyway, they proved that the combined use of DM, DBT, and US provided sensitivity and accuracy results (98 % and 94 %, respectively) comparable to the ones achieved by breast MRI alone (99 % and 92 %). The use of tomosynthesis added to conventional techniques (mammography and ultrasound) proved to be highly reliable for preoperative staging of breast cancer and to match the performances usually achieved by breast MRI (Mariscotti et al. 2014). Nonetheless, Mariscotti and colleagues reported that the sensitivity of MRI in preoperative assessment was not significantly affected in dense breasts (98 %), but it was reduced for mammography and tomosynthesis (79 % and 87 %, respectively) instead (Mariscotti et al. 2014). The role of US added to mammography and DBT in dense breasts was not studied by Mariscotti and colleagues, but the highest sensitivity (92 %) showed by US alone could be probably positively affect the diagnostic performances of mammography and tomosynthesis, as previously described (Elizalde et al. 2014; Kim et al. 2015).

- *In preoperative setting, breast MRI shows the best sensitivity particularly for detection of multifocal/multicentric disease and for invasive lobular carcinoma.*
- *In cases in which breast MRI is not feasible or not indicated, the complementary use of digital mammography, digital breast tomosynthesis, and ultrasound proved to have a diagnostic accuracy comparable to MRI.*

- *Lesion's diameters measured on tomosynthetic images are more accurate and concordant with the pathological result than diameters measured on mammography.*

## 4.4 Digital Breast Tomosynthesis as "Second-Look" Technique After Breast Magnetic Resonance Imaging

Breast MRI is the most sensitive imaging method for the detection of breast cancer (Warner et al. 2008; Houssami et al. 2008). Therefore, additional breast lesions that have not been previously detected by conventional imaging (mammography and US) could be identified at a breast MRI examination. In a preoperative setting, lesions detected at breast MRI and rated as suspicious need to be sampled at biopsy for pathologic verification. Although MRI-guided biopsy is a safe and accurate diagnostic tool, its broad application is limited by its costs, availability, and requirement for contrast medium administration (Floery and Helbich 2006; Perlet et al. 2006). Typically, a correct management of these new diagnosed lesions at breast MRI implies a new targeted ultrasound evaluation of them, guided by MRI imaging, known by the name of "second-look US". The primary role of second-look US is to support decision making in clinical practice by helping locate the MRI-detected lesion and obtaining pathological verification with US-guided instead of MRI-guided biopsy. Ultrasound-guided biopsies are, in general, desirable as they are less costly, more broadly available, and more comfortable for the patient (Leung 2011). A recent meta-analysis on the diagnostic utility of second-look US, which included benign and malignant lesions evaluated in seventeen studies, showed a very heterogeneous general lesion detection (between 22.6 % and 82.1 %) with a pooled rate of 57.5 % (Spick and Baltzer 2014). The highest second-look US detection rates were observed for mass lesions (66 %, as opposed to a 29 % of non-mass lesions) and malignant (79 % versus 52 % of benign) lesions ($p<0.001$ for both). Pooled positive and negative predictive values (positive or negative second-look US correlates with MRI-detected malignant or benign lesions) were calculated as 30.7 % and 87.8 %, respectively (Spick and Baltzer 2014). These results showed that not all newly diagnosed MRI lesions and, more importantly, not all malignant lesions could be detected by second-look US. Two studies (Clauser et al. 2015, Mariscotti 2015) evaluated the role of "second-look" digital breast tomosynthesis and its use to detect newly diagnosed lesions at preoperative breast MRI. Clauser and colleagues evaluated 135 patients who underwent breast MRI examination for preoperative evaluation after a diagnosis of breast cancer at conventional imaging (DM, US, percutaneous biopsy with histological examination). MR images revealed 84 newly diagnosed lesions categorized as BI-RADS 3 (probably benign), BI-RADS 4 (suspicious), or BI-RADS 5 (highly suspicious) according to BI-RADS lexicon (D'Orsi et al. 2013), detected in 53/135 patients (39 %). At second-look US, a correlate was found for 44/84 (52 %) lesions, similarly to results showed by the meta-analysis of Spick and colleagues (2014). Second-look DBT detected 42/84 (50 %) lesions, almost the same number as second-look US, but not the same lesions. In fact, 19/84

(23 %) lesions were detected by second-look DBT only, for a total of 63/84 (75 %) newly diagnosed MRI lesions detected by second-look examination (US or DBT) (Clauser et al. 2015). According to the authors, the contribution of second-look DBT was relevant in particular for non-mass findings. In fact, the increase was from 64 % to 86 % (+22 %) for mass findings, while it was between 28 % and 61 % (+33 %) for non-mass findings. This means that in adding second-look DBT to second-look US, the detection rate of mass findings went up to nearly 90 %, while the rate of non-mass findings reached only around 60 % (but second-look DBT enabled the detection of one-third of non-mass findings not detected by second-look US). This aspect can also be appreciated looking at pathology: of seven ductal carcinomas in situ, four were detected at second-look DBT, and none at second-look US. Conversely, of 11 invasive lobular carcinomas, eight were detected at second-look US and only two at second-look DBT. This shows the complementary role of these two approaches in the detection of different cancer types, also considering that non-mass MRI findings presented at DBT as subtle microcalcifications or focal asymmetries are usually very difficult to detect using US. Notably, only 20 out of 42 second-look DBT detected lesions were detected at a second-look mammography (Clauser et al. 2015). These results seem to confirm the lower detection rate of second-look mammography (6 % for all lesions and 19 % for non-mass lesions) showed by Trop and colleagues when compared to second-look US (Trop et al. 2010) and they could be partially explained by the limited mammographic accuracy in dense breasts. Anyway, Clauser and colleagues did not find any significant differences when considering the presence of a correlate at second-look DBT and breast density (Clauser et al. 2015).

Mariscotti and colleagues evaluated 164 MRI newly detected lesions (in 114/520 women, 22 %) with a second-look imaging; second-look US identified 114/164 (70 %) of these, whereas 50/164 (30 %) remained unidentified (Mariscotti et al. 2015). Second-look DBT identified 32/50 of these cases, increasing the overall characterization of MRI-detected additional findings to 89.0 % (146/164) (Mariscotti et al. 2015). As showed by Clauser and colleagues (2015), a correlation at tomosynthesis was significantly more frequent for non-mass enhancement lesions ($p = 0.02$) (Mariscotti et al. 2015). This underlines the complementary role of second-look DBT to second-look US, more reliable in detecting mass-type lesions found at MRI (Spick and Baltzer 2014). Furthermore, compared to second-look US, second-look DBT can be performed while looking at MRI images even before recalling the patient, thus giving more diagnostic information before the patient eventually returns for second-look US; even more, tomosynthesis is very likely less operator dependent, and more than one radiologist, when necessary, can review the images.

Interestingly, Mariscotti and colleagues showed the utility of a sort of "third-look US" (a repeated second-look US targeted to correlated MRI and DBT findings), which allowed identification of 24/32 (75 %) corresponding US abnormalities unseen at the initial second-look US MRI guided only. Consequently, US-guided needle biopsy was possible in most of these cases, taking advantage of rapidity and easiness, and acceptability to patients, of this technique (Mariscotti et al. 2015).

These papers about the role of second-look DBT showed different results about the rate of malignancy in MRI additional lesions occult at both second-look US and second-look DBT, respectively, 17/21 (81 %) (Clauser et al. 2015) and 1/18 (6 %) (Mariscotti et al. 2015). Compared to not visualized lesions at second-look US, for which malignancy might occur in a pooled estimate of about 12 % (Spick and Baltzer 2014), these results appear to be over- and underestimated, respectively. The reason should be probably related to the inclusion criteria in preoperative MRI patients; in fact Clauser and colleagues selected a higher number of multifocal/ multicentric breast cancers, as proved by the higher rate of women with additional lesions at MRI (53/135, 39 %) and ipsilateral lesions (67/84, 80 %) (Clauser et al. 2015) compared to respective rates in the population of Mariscotti and colleagues for women with additional lesions (114/520 women, 22 %) and ipsilateral findings (32/50, 68 % of lesions found at second-look DBT) (Mariscotti et al. 2015). Anyway, both results proved that additional findings detected at breast MRI which do not have any second-look US or DBT correlate deserve MR-guided biopsy, unless very close to a lesion already proven to be malignant (thus allowing for a relatively easy surgical removal) (Leung 2011; Luciani et al. 2011; Spick and Baltzer 2014).

Regarding the possibility to perform a biopsy of findings detected at second-look DBT, the introduction of methods for biopsy under DBT guidance (Dershaw 2013; Viala et al. 2013) proved to be a safe and effective procedure. It is usually performed using a full-field DM system equipped with a three-dimensional tomosynthesis platform (Selenia Dimensions 3D; Hologic, was the first system used by these authors (Dershaw 2013; Viala et al. 2013; Schrading et al. 2015)). For breast biopsy, a dedicated guidance must be installed as an add-on, and it could be used for "conventional," two-dimensional mammography-guided stereotactic breast biopsy or it can be used in DBT mode for DBT-guided biopsy. The patient can be positioned in a lateral decubitus or sitting position (chosen on the basis of the lesion location) on a dedicated armchair. The breast must be fixated with a special compression paddle, and DBT should be performed to reidentify the target lesion. The biopsy coordinates, including z-axis location, are determined directly from the DBT images by identifying the DBT section that yielded the sharpest depiction of the target. Coordinates are automatically determined by the biopsy software system after the operator indicated the position of the target with a cursor. The vacuum-assisted biopsy (VAB) procedure is identical to the procedure performed by using any common stereotactic-guided system; even pre- and post-fire control images are usually obtained by using a pair of stereotactic full-field digital mammographic images, because the inserted needle would lead to artifacts at DBT. After the biopsy, postbiopsy control can be performed using DBT (Schrading et al. 2015).

Schrading and colleagues compared 51 DBT-guided VABs with 165 stereotactic-guided VABs and showed that reidentifying and retargeting lesions during stereotactic-guided VABs took longer than it did during DBT-guided VABs ($p<0.001$), while the tissue sampling took about the same time for both procedures ($p=0.067$). The lesions were successfully identified and biopsied on all (51/51) examinations, and the only complications occurred were vasovagal reactions, more common in the sitting position (Schrading et al. 2015).

Though DBT-guided biopsy implies radiation exposure (lower than that needed for stereotactic mammographic guidance (Viala et al. 2013), anyway), the lack of contrast agent injection and the good technical success described by initial experiences proved this technique to be faster and more comfortable for the patient compared to MRI-guided biopsy. Furthermore, the availability of a DBT-guided needle localization has proved to be a useful tool in DBT-detected suspicious abnormalities not visualized with other modalities in the preoperative setting (Freer et al. 2015).

- *Digital breast tomosynthesis is a feasible and sensitive "second-look" approach for the identification of additional findings at preoperative MRI, and it is complementary to "second-look" ultrasound.*
- *The availability of DBT-guided vacuum-assisted biopsies and preoperative needle localizations can be faster and more comfortable for the patient than MRI-guided or standard mammography-guided procedures.*

## References

ACR Guidelines and Standards Committee, Basset LW, Berg WA, Birdwell RL et al (2008) ACR practice guideline for the performance of contrast-enhanced magnetic resonance imaging (MRI) of the breast. Available via http://www.acr.org/SecondaryMainMenuCategories/quality_safety/guidelines/breast/mri_breast.aspx

Althuis MD, Dozier JM, Anderson WF, Devesa SS, Brinton LA (2005) Global trends in breast cancer incidence and mortality 1973–1997. Int J Epidemiol 34(2):405–412

Andersson I, Ikeda DM, Zackrisson S, Ruschin M, Svahn T, Timberg P, Tingberg A (2008) Breast tomosynthesis and digital mammography: a comparison of breast cancer visibility and BIRADS classification in a population of cancers with subtle mammographic findings. Eur Radiol 18(12):2817–2825

Brandt KR, Craig DA, Hoskins TL, Henrichsen TL, Bendel EC, Brandt SR, Mandrekar J (2013) Can digital breast tomosynthesis replace conventional diagnostic mammography views for screening recalls without calcifications? A comparison study in a simulated clinical setting. AJR Am J Roentgenol 200(2):291–298

Ciatto S, Houssami N, Bernardi D, Caumo F, Pellegrini M, Brunelli S, Tuttobene P, Bricolo P, Fantò C, Valentini M, Montemezzi S, Macaskill P (2013) Integration of 3D digital mammography with tomosynthesis for population breast-cancer screening (STORM): a prospective comparison study. Lancet Oncol 14(7):583–589

Clauser P, Carbonaro LA, Pancot M, Girometti R, Bazzocchi M, Zuiani C, Sardanelli F (2015) Additional findings at preoperative breast MRI: the value of second-look digital breast tomosynthesis. Eur Radiol 25:2830–2839

Cohen Y (2014) Tomosynthesis assisting in localization of breast lesions for ultrasound targeting seen on one mammographic view only. AJR Am J Roentgenol 203(5):W555

D'Orsi CJ, Sickles EA, Mendelson EB, Morris EA (2013) Breast imaging and reporting data system: ACR BI-RADS breast imaging atlas. American College of Radiology, Reston

Dershaw DD (2013) Large core needle biopsy with tomosynthesis guidance: another development in breast imaging technology. Breast J 19(1):1–3

Elizalde A, Pina L, Etxano J, Slon P, Zalazar R, Caballeros M (2016) Additional US or DBT after digital mammography: which one is the best combination? Acta Radiol 57(1):13–8

ElMaadawy MM, Seely JM, Doherty G, Lad SV (2012) Digital breast tomosynthesis in the evaluation of focal mammographic asymmetry: do you still need coned compression views? [abstr].

In: Radiological Society of North America Scientific Assembly and Annual Meeting Program. Radiological Society of North America, Oak Brook, p 158

Floery D, Helbich TH (2006) MRI-guided percutaneous biopsy of breast lesions: materials, techniques, success rates, and management in patients with suspected radiologic-pathologic mismatch [viii.]. Magn Reson Imaging Clin N Am 14(3):411–425, viii

Förnvik D, Zackrisson S, Ljungberg O, Svahn T, Timberg P, Tingberg A, Andersson I (2010) Breast tomosynthesis: accuracy of tumor measurement compared with digital mammography and ultrasonography. Acta Radiol 51(3):240–247

Freer PE, Niell B, Rafferty EA (2015) Preoperative tomosynthesis-guided needle localization of mammographically and sonographically occult breast lesions. Radiology 275(2):377–383

Girardi V, Tonegutti M, Ciatto S, Bonetti F (2013) Breast ultrasound in 22,131 asymptomatic women with negative mammography. Breast 22(5):806–809

Gur D, Abrams GS, Chough DM et al (2009) Digital breast tomosynthesis: observer performance study. AJR Am J Roentgenol 193:586–591

Harvey JA, Nicholson BT, Cohen MA (2008) Finding early invasive breast cancers: a practical approach. Radiology 248(1):61–76

Houssami N, Ciatto S, Macaskill P, Lord SJ, Warren RM, Dixon JM, Irwig L (2008) Accuracy and surgical impact of magnetic resonance imaging in breast cancer staging: systematic review and meta-analysis in detection of multifocal and multicentric cancer. J Clin Oncol 26(19):3248–3258

Kim MJ, Kim EK, Kwak JY, Son EJ, Youk JH, Choi SH, Han M, Oh KK (2009) Characterization of microcalcification: can digital monitor zooming replace magnification mammography in full-field digital mammography? Eur Radiol 19(2):310–317

Kim SA, Chang JM, Cho N, Yi A, Moon WK (2015) Characterization of breast lesions: comparison of digital breast tomosynthesis and ultrasonography. Korean J Radiol 16(2):229–238

Kopans D, Gavenonis S, Halpern E, Moore R (2011) Calcifications in the breast and digital breast tomosynthesis. Breast J 17(6):638–644

Leung JW (2011) Utility of second-look ultrasound in the evaluation of MRI-detected breast lesions. Semin Roentgenol 46(4):260–274

Luciani ML, Pediconi F, Telesca M, Vasselli F, Casali V, Miglio E, Passariello R, Catalano C (2011) Incidental enhancing lesions found on preoperative breast MRI: management and role of second-look ultrasound. Radiol Med 116(6):886–904

Luparia A, Mariscotti G, Durando M, Ciatto S, Bosco D, Campanino PP, Castellano I, Sapino A, Gandini G (2013) Accuracy of tumour size assessment in the preoperative staging of breast cancer: comparison of digital mammography, tomosynthesis, ultrasound and MRI. Radiol Med 118(7):1119–1136

Mann RM, Kuhl CK, Kinkel K, Boetes C (2008a) Breast MRI: guidelines from the European Society of Breast Imaging. Eur Radiol 18(7):1307–1318

Mann RM, Veltman J, Barentsz JO, Wobbes T, Blickman JG, Boetes C (2008b) The value of MRI compared to mammography in the assessment of tumour extent in invasive lobular carcinoma of the breast. Eur J Surg Oncol 34(2):135–142

Mariscotti G, Houssami N, Durando M, Bergamasco L, Campanino PP, Ruggieri C, Regini E, Luparia A, Bussone R, Sapino A, Fonio P, Gandini G (2014) Accuracy of mammography, digital breast tomosynthesis, ultrasound and MR imaging in preoperative assessment of breast cancer. Anticancer Res 34(3):1219–1225, PubMed

Mariscotti G, Houssami N, Durando M, Campanino PP, Regini E, Fornari A, Bussone R, Castellano I, Sapino A, Fonio P, Gandini G (2015) Digital breast tomosynthesis (DBT) to characterize MRI-detected additional lesions unidentified at targeted ultrasound in newly diagnosed breast cancer patients. Eur Radiol 25:2673–2681

Mun HS, Kim HH, Shin HJ, Cha JH, Ruppel PL, Oh HY, Chae EY (2013) Assessment of extent of breast cancer: comparison between digital breast tomosynthesis and full-field digital mammography. Clin Radiol 68(12):1254–1259

Niklason LT, Christian BT, Niklason LE, Kopans DB, Castleberry DE, Opsahl-Ong BH, Landberg CE, Slanetz PJ, Giardino AA, Moore R, Albagli D, DeJule MC, Fitzgerald PF, Fobare DF, Giambattista BW, Kwasnick RF, Liu J, Lubowski SJ, Possin GE, Richotte JF, Wei CY, Wirth RF (1997) Digital tomosynthesis in breast imaging. Radiology 205(2):399–406

Noroozian M, Hadjiiski L, Rahnama-Moghadam S, Klein KA, Jeffries DO, Pinsky RW, Chan HP, Carson PL, Helvie MA, Roubidoux MA (2012) Digital breast tomosynthesis is comparable to mammographic spot views for mass characterization. Radiology 262(1):61–68

Orvieto E, Maiorano E, Bottiglieri L, Maisonneuve P, Rotmensz N, Galimberti V, Luini A, Brenelli F, Gatti G, Viale G (2008) Clinicopathologic characteristics of invasive lobular carcinoma of the breast: results of an analysis of 530 cases from a single institution. Cancer 113(7):1511–1520

Peppard HR, Nicholson BE, Rochman CM, Merchant JK, Mayo RC 3rd, Harvey JA (2015) Digital breast tomosynthesis in the diagnostic setting: indications and clinical applications. Radiographics 35:975–990

Perlet C, Heywang-Kobrunner SH, Heinig A et al (2006) Magnetic resonance-guided, vacuum-assisted breast biopsy: results from a European multicenter study of 538 lesions. Cancer 106(5):982–990

Sardanelli F, Boetes C, Borisch B, Decker T, Federico M, Gilbert FJ, Helbich T, Heywang-Köbrunner SH, Kaiser WA, Kerin MJ, Mansel RE, Marotti L, Martincich L, Mauriac L, Meijers-Heijboer H, Orecchia R, Panizza P, Ponti A, Purushotham AD, Regitnig P, Del Turco MR, Thibault F, Wilson R (2010) Magnetic resonance imaging of the breast: recommendations from the EUSOMA working group. Eur J Cancer 46(8):1296–1316

Schrading S, Distelmaier M, Dirrichs T, Detering S, Brolund L, Strobel K, Kuhl CK (2015) Digital breast tomosynthesis-guided vacuum-assisted breast biopsy: initial experiences and comparison with prone stereotactic vacuum-assisted biopsy. Radiology 274(3):654–662

Sickles EA (1989) Combining spot-compression and other special views to maximize mammographic information. Radiology 173:571

Skaane P, Bandos AI, Gullien R, Eben EB, Ekseth U, Haakenaasen U, Izadi M, Jebsen IN, Jahr G, Krager M, Niklason LT, Hofvind S, Gur D (2013) Comparison of digital mammography alone and digital mammography plus tomosynthesis in a population-based screening program. Radiology 267(1):47–56

Spangler ML, Zuley ML, Sumkin JH, Abrams G, Ganott MA, Hakim C, Perrin R, Chough DM, Shah R, Gur D (2011) Detection and classification of calcifications on digital breast tomosynthesis and 2D digital mammography: a comparison. AJR Am J Roentgenol 196(2):320–324. doi:10.2214/AJR.10.4656, Erratum in: AJR Am J Roentgenol. 2011 Mar;196(3):743

Spick C, Baltzer PA (2014) Diagnostic utility of second-look US for breast lesions identified at MR imaging: systematic review and meta-analysis. Radiology 273(2):401–409

Tagliafico A, Astengo D, Cavagnetto F, Rosasco R, Rescinito G, Monetti F, Calabrese M (2012) One-to-one comparison between digital spot compression view and digital breast tomosynthesis. Eur Radiol 22(3):539–544

Tagliafico A, Mariscotti G, Durando M, Stevanin C, Tagliafico G, Martino L, Bignotti B, Calabrese M, Houssami N (2015) Characterisation of microcalcification clusters on 2D digital mammography (FFDM) and digital breast tomosynthesis (DBT): does DBT underestimate microcalcification clusters? Results of a multicenter study. Eur Radiol 25(1):9–14

Trop I, Labelle M, David J, Mayrand MH, Lalonde L (2010) Second-look targeted studies after breast magnetic resonance imaging: practical tips to improve lesion identification. Curr Probl Diagn Radiol 39(5):200–211

Viala J, Gignier P, Perret B, Hovasse C, Hovasse D, Chancelier-Galan MD, Bornet G, Hamrouni A, Lasry JL, Convard JP (2013) Stereotactic vacuum-assisted biopsies on a digital breast 3D-tomosynthesis system. Breast J 19(1):4–9

Warner E, Messersmith H, Causer P, Eisen A, Shumak R, Plewes D (2008) Systematic review: using magnetic resonance imaging to screen women at high risk for breast cancer. Ann Intern Med 148(9):671–679

Zuley ML, Bandos AI, Ganott MA, Sumkin JH, Kelly AE, Catullo VJ, Rathfon GY, Lu AH, Gur D (2013) Digital breast tomosynthesis versus supplemental diagnostic mammographic views for evaluation of noncalcified breast lesions. Radiology 266(1):89–95

# Clinical Cases

# 5

Massimo Calabrese, Sonia Airaldi, Lucia Martino,
Bianca Bignotti, Licia Gristina, Giovanna Mariscotti,
Manuela Durando, Davide Astengo, and Alberto Tagliafico

**Electronic supplementary material** The online version of this chapter (doi:10.1007/978-3-319-28631-0_5) contains supplementary material, which is available to authorized users.

M. Calabrese (✉)
Senologia Diagnostica e Diagnostica per Immagini IRCCS Azienda Ospedaliera
Universitaria San Martino – Ist Istituto Nazionale per la Ricerca sul Cancro,
Largo Rosanna Benzi, 10, Genova 16132, Italy
e-mail: massimo.calabrese@hsanmartino.it; maxcala@virgilio.it

S. Airaldi, MD • L. Martino, MD • B. Bignotti, MD • L. Gristina, MD • D. Astengo, MD
Department of Health Sciences, University of Genova, Genova, Italy
e-mail: airaldi.sonia@gmail.com; luci.84@hotmail.it; bignottibianca@gmail.com;
licia.gristina@virgilio.it; davide7412@yahoo.it

G. Mariscotti • M. Durando
Department of Diagnostic Imaging and Radiotherapy, Radiology University of Torino,
Azienda Ospedaliero-Universitaria, Città della Salute e della Scienza di Torino
Via Genova 3, Torino 10126, Italy
e-mail: giovanna.mariscotti@libero.it; mdurando@cittadellasalute.to.it

A. Tagliafico
Department of Experimental Medicine, DIMES- Institute of Anatomy
University of Genova, Via de Toni 14, Genova 16132, Italy
e-mail: alberto.tagliafico@unige.it; albertotagliafico@gmail.com;
http://www.albertotagliafico.com

© Springer International Publishing Switzerland 2016
A. Tagliafico et al. (eds.), *Digital Breast Tomosynthesis: A Practical Approach*,
DOI 10.1007/978-3-319-28631-0_5

## Abbreviations

| | |
|---|---|
| CC | Craniocaudal |
| DBT | Digital breast tomosynthesis |
| EUSOBI | European Society of Breast Imaging |
| EUSOMA | European Society of Breast Cancer Specialists |
| FFDM | Full-field digital mammography |
| MIP | Maximum intensity projection |
| MLO | Mediolateral oblique |
| MRI | Magnetic resonance imaging |
| SIRM | Società Italiana di Radiologia Medica |
| US | Ultrasound |

In this chapter, our purpose is to show some cases that may occur in daily clinical practice. We included mainly screening cases. In Italy there is a lot of spontaneous screening accompanied by an organized population-based screening. The use of ultrasound is widely adopted especially in women with dense breast and in young women. Radiologists perform ultrasound and have specific breast ultrasound screening expertise. Ultrasound is also used for second look after MRI. The use of DBT for second look after MRI is still under evaluation, although a promising research on 520 patients (Mariscotti et al. 2015) found that DBT was able to identify a further 32 of the 50 lesions unidentified on targeted US after MRI. DBT improved the characterization of additional MR findings and may have the potential to improve breast cancer staging. The radiologists who provided the cases have a proven track record of at least 5000 mammograms per annum, DBT usage since 2009, and clinical and screening US usage with a minimum of 7 years of experience in breast imaging. The radiologists who provided the cases work following EUSOMA, EUSOBI, and SIRM guidelines and recommendations.

The radiologists who provided these cases are among the first who published in Italy a clinical study, highly cited, on the usefulness of DBT in clinical setting (Tagliafico et al. 2012). Most DBT images were read using Hologic SecurView DW workstations, optimized to read both FFDM and TS images.

The images presented on tomosynthesis are completed with the corresponding video clips in the online version. We hope that this case presentation will help, especially beginners, in understanding the potential and limitation of DBT compared to mammography, US, and MRI.

Each case can be read as a stand-alone presentation and some of them are presented including take-home messages. Others are presented to let the reader gain experience on DBT images and videos. We decided not to insert the BI-RADS classification due to the known discrepancies between the USA and Europe in its use and due to the reduced intra- and interobserver agreement.

## References

Mariscotti G, Houssami N, Durando M, Campanino PP, Regini E, Fornari A, Bussone R, Castellano I, Sapino A, Fonio P, Gandini G (2015) Digital breast tomosynthesis (DBT) to characterize MRI-detected additional lesions unidentified at targeted ultrasound in newly diagnosed breast cancer patients. Eur Radiol 25(9):2673–2681. doi: 10.1007/s00330-015-3669-4. Epub 2015 Mar 27

Tagliafico A, Astengo D, Cavagnetto F, Rosasco R, Rescinito G, Monetti F, Calabrese M (2012) One-to-one comparison between digital spot compression view and digital breast tomosynthesis. Eur Radiol 22(3):539–544. doi: 10.1007/s00330-011-2305-1. Epub 2011 Oct 11

## 5.1    Case Presentations

### 5.1.1    Case 1

**Case History**  Woman, 71 years old, underwent mammography for screening purposes. She reported no symptoms and the family history was unremarkable.

**Standard Mammography**  Heterogeneously dense breast. Screening craniocaudal FFDM image depicts an architectural distortion (*white arrow*) in the lateral middle third of the right breast. No further suspicious findings are present.

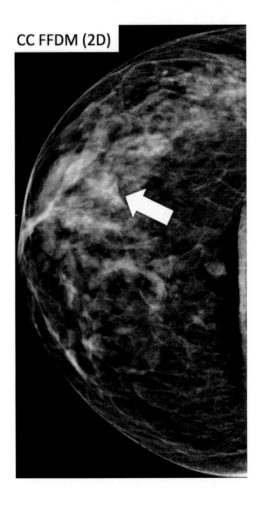

**Tomosynthesis** Left craniocaudal DBT image shows normal findings. The suspicious architectural distortion shown on mammography is considered not visible (*white circle*). Therefore, DBT solved the suspicious mammographic finding.

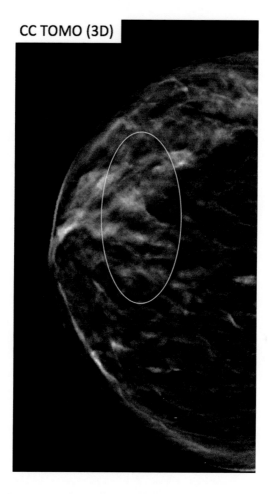

**Conclusion** In this case, DBT solved suspicious mammographic finding avoiding a biopsy. The distortion seen on FFDM was caused by tissue superimposition. No recall was necessary (See Video C1c).

## 5.1.2   Case 2

**Case History**   Woman, 55 years old, underwent mammography for screening purposes. She reported no symptoms and the family history was unremarkable.

**Standard Mammography**   Scattered areas of fibroglandular density breast. Left craniocaudal and mediolateral oblique FFDM images show an equal-density irregular mass with indistinct margin (*arrowhead*) and cluster of microcalcifications (*white arrow*) in the central middle third of the superior left breast.

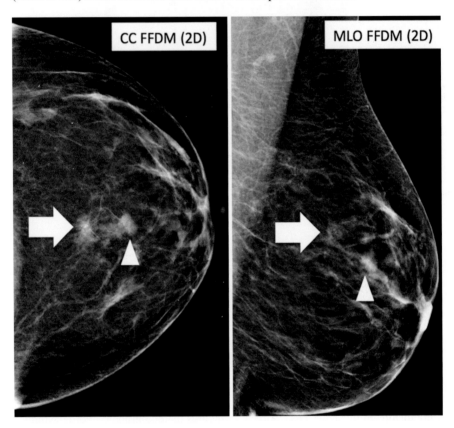

**Tomosynthesis** Left craniocaudal and mediolateral oblique DBT images support mammographic finding. DBT images show the suspicious mass (*arrowhead*) and demonstrate the cluster of microcalcifications (*white arrow*) in the middle third of the superior left breast. However, on DBT, the cluster of microcalcifications was scored less suspicious than on MX and it was less visible.

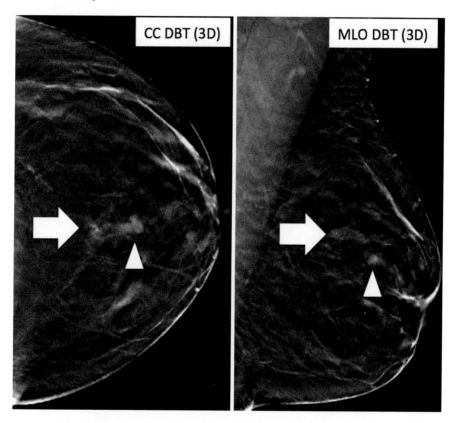

**Conclusions** Tomosynthesis supports mammographic findings, but the detection of microcalcifications was worst (lower number of micro detected) than on FFDM, probably due to lack of superimposed tissue. Final diagnosis was ductal carcinoma with in situ components (See Videos C2_LCC and C2_LMLO).

## References

Tagliafico A, Houssami N (2015) Digital breast tomosynthesis might not be the optimal modality for detecting microcalcification. Radiology 275(2):618–619. doi: 10.1148/radiol.2015142752

Tagliafico A, Mariscotti G, Durando M et al (2014) Characterization of microcalcification clusters on 2D digital mammography (FFDM) and digital breast tomosynthesis (DBT): does DBT underestimate microcalcification clusters? Results of a multicentre study. Eur Radiol. 2015;25(1):9–14. doi: 10.1007/s00330-014-3402-8. Epub 2014 Aug 29.

### 5.1.3  Case 3

**Case History**  Woman, 55 years old, underwent mammography for screening purposes. No symptoms, family history unremarkable.

**Standard Mammography**  Extremely dense breast. Right MLO FFDM image shows a suspicious mass (*white arrow*) with associated calcifications and fat in upper outer quadrant. No further suspicious findings are present.

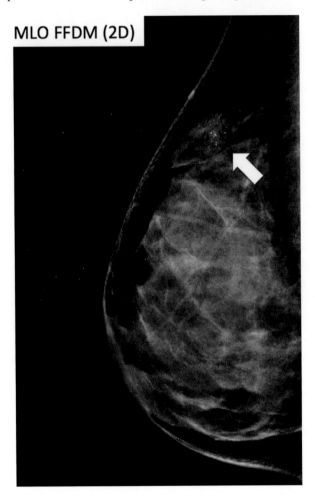

**Tomosynthesis** DBT confirms the presence of a mass with associated microcalcifications (*white circle*) and fat. Therefore, DBT confirmed the suspicious mammographic finding.

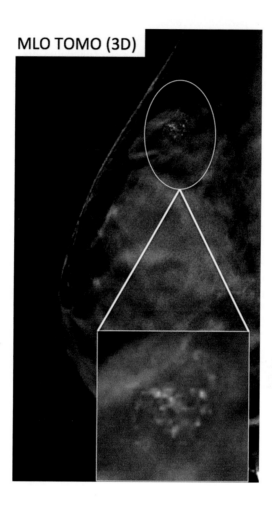

**Conclusion** The result of the histological exam was ductal carcinoma in situ, (DCIS) so in this case, DBT confirmed the suspicious mammographic finding (See Video C3).

The mass is only partially circumscribed and contains fat, and it seems not completely encapsulated. Several masses may contain fat which is radiolucent at DBT. Most encapsulated fat-containing masses (including lipomas, hamartomas, galactoceles, and lipid cysts) are benign; nonencapsulated fat-containing masses (especially spiculated fat-containing masses) are considered malignant (Freer et al. 2014) until proven otherwise.

Masses seen at DBT should be evaluated according to their shape and margins rather than their fat content, and the presence of fat is not sufficient to avoid biopsy (Peppard et al. 2015).

## Reference

Freer PE, Wang JL, Rafferty EA (2014) Digital breast tomosynthesis in the analysis of fat-containing lesions. RadioGraphics 34(2):343–358. 2

Peppard HR, Nicholson BE, Rochman CM, Merchant JK, Mayo RC 3rd, Harvey JA (2015) Digital breast tomosynthesis in the diagnostic setting: indications and clinical applications. Radiographics 35(4):975–990. doi: 10.1148/rg.2015140204. Epub 2015 May 29

### 5.1.4   Case 4

**Case History** Woman, 82 years old, underwent tomosynthesis and ultrasound examination to evaluate suspicious finding in the right breast. The lesion was palpable.

FFDM not shown.

**Tomosynthesis** Right MLO DBT image shows a high-density irregular mass in the middle third of the right breast (*white arrow*), approximately 30 mm in diameter, with associated nipple and skin retraction.

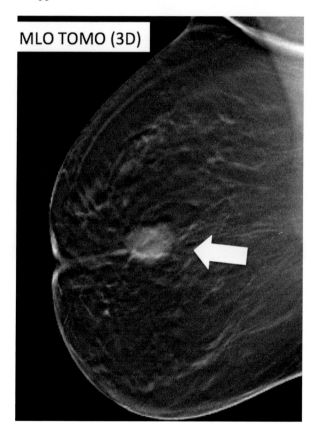

**Ultrasound** Corresponding US image demonstrates an irregular mass with spiculated margins and posterior acoustic shadowing in the right breast at 12 o'clock
position. Therefore, the high-suspicious lesion is also visible at ultrasound, but the
measured diameter was 20 mm. Biopsy confirmed a B5b lesion (invasive lobular
carcinoma).

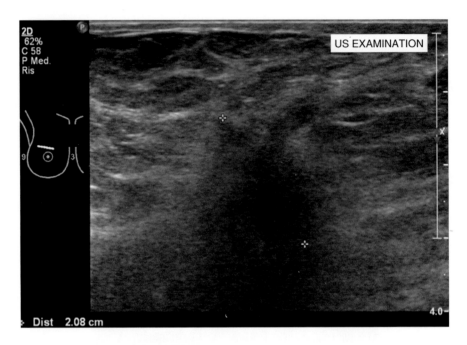

**Conclusions** Tomosynthesis allowed a better evaluation (staging) of the lesion
because at pathology the lesion was 32 mm.

> "DBT and MRI are superior to DM and US in the preoperative assessment of breast tumor
> size. DBT seems to improve the accuracy of DM, although MRI remains the most accurate
> imaging modality for breast cancer extension by Luparia et al."

# Reference

Luparia A, Mariscotti G, Durando M, Ciatto S, Bosco D, Campanino PP, Castellano I,
Sapino A, Gandini G (2013) Accuracy of tumor size assessment in the preoperative
staging of breast cancer: comparison of digital mammography, tomosynthesis,
ultrasound and MRI. Radiol Med 118(7):1119–1136. doi: 10.1007/s11547-013-
0941-z. Epub 2013 Jun 25

### 5.1.5   Case 5

**Case History** Woman, 72 years old, underwent tomosynthesis and ultrasound examination to evaluate suspicious finding in the right breast visible only on CC DBT. FFDM not shown and negative.

**Tomosynthesis** Right CC DBT image shows a small architectural distortion/mass (*white arrow*) in posterior third of the medial right breast (approximately 4 mm) with a radiolucent core. This is a suspicious finding and it was considered worthy of further evaluation.

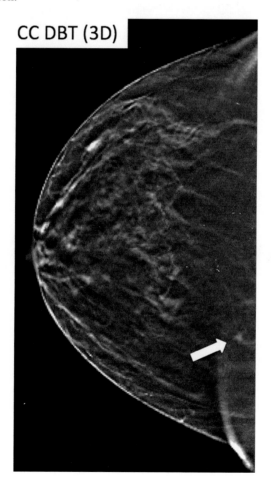

Ultrasound examination was negative.

Stereotactic VABB of the small architectural distortion at inner quadrants (*white arrow*) gave the following result: B5b, invasive ductal carcinoma.

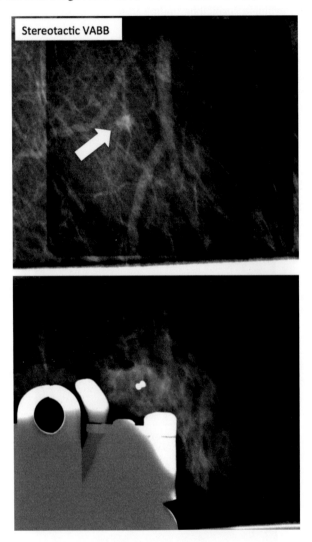

**Conclusions** DBT allowed depiction of a lesion not visible at FFDM (and at US in this case) (See Video C5).

## 5.1.6 Case 6

**Case History** Woman, 62 years old, underwent tomosynthesis and ultrasound examination to evaluate suspicious finding in the left breast. FFDM not shown.

**Tomosynthesis** Left CC and MLO DBT image show an architectural distortion (*white circle*) located in the upper inner quadrant.

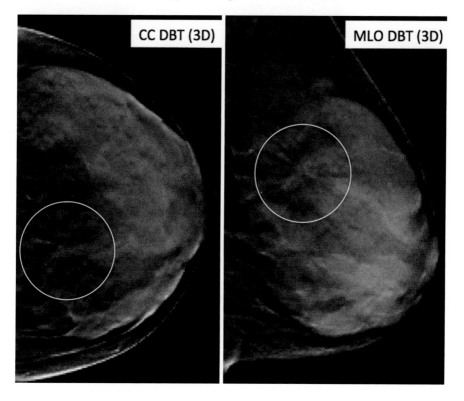

**Ultrasound** Corresponding US image demonstrates a 6-mm hypoechoic mass with indistinct margins at 10 o'clock position in the upper inner quadrant of the left breast.

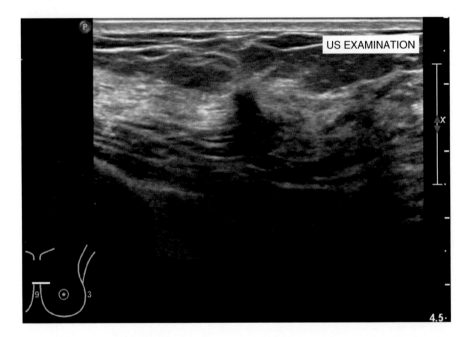

US-guided core needle biopsy demonstrated a B5b lesion (invasive ductal carcinoma).

**MRI** MRI evaluation confirmed the presence of a mass (10 mm) in the upper inner quadrant of the left breast (*white arrow*). No metastatic lymphadenopathy in the axillary region. No masses in the contralateral breast. (**a**) Postcontrast subtracted image. (**b**) Postcontrast maximum intensity projection image.

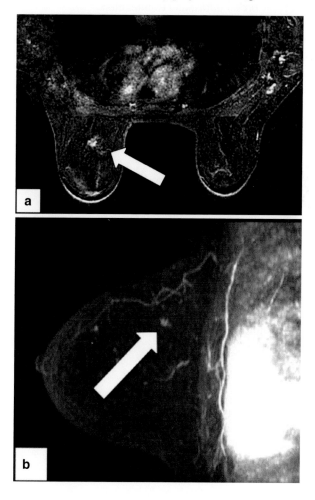

**Conclusions** DBT allowed a good evaluation of the architectural distortion (See Videos C6_LCC and C6_LMLO).

### 5.1.7 Case 7

**Case History** Woman, 73 years old, underwent tomosynthesis and ultrasound-guided biopsy for staging purposes. A small mass (5 mm) in the left breast was detected in a previous breast ultrasound examination.

**Tomosynthesis** Left CC DBT image shows an irregular mass with indistinct margins in the central breast (*white arrow*).

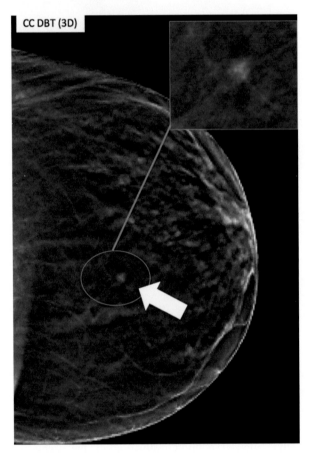

**Ultrasound** Corresponding US image shows a suspicious hyperechoic mass, approximately 7 mm with indistinct margins, in the left breast at 12 o'clock position (*white arrow*).

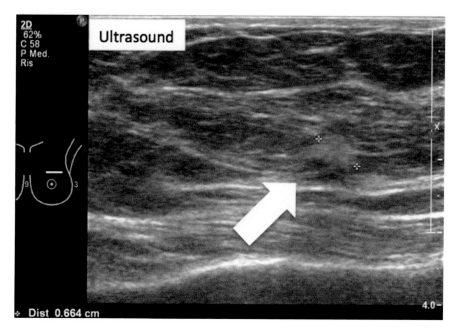

The US-guided core needle biopsy confirmed a B5b lesion (invasive lobular carcinoma).

**MRI**  MRI evaluation confirms the presence of the lesion (6 mm) in the left breast (*white arrow*) and shows an in situ component of 25 mm. No metastatic lymphadenopathy in the axillary region.

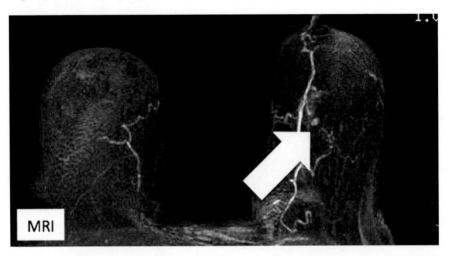

**Conclusions**  DBT allowed a good evaluation of the margins of the lesion, but MRI was better for staging (See Video C7_LCC).

## 5.1.8   Case 8

**Case History**   Woman, 52 years old, who underwent mammography for screening purposes. No symptoms and no palpable lumps at clinical examination.

**Mammography**   Heterogeneously dense breast. Right MLO FFDM image shows an area of architectural distortion (*white arrow*) in the posterior third of the superior right breast. No further suspicious findings.

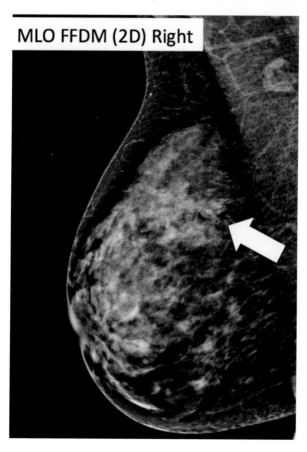

MLO FFDM (2D) Right

**Tomosynthesis** Right MLO DBT image confirms the presence of architectural distortion in the posterior third of the superior right breast (*white arrow*). DBT allows improved visualization of the architectural distortion.

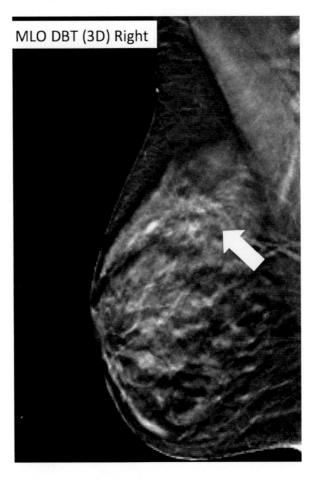

**Ultrasound**  No suspicious findings are detected in the *right breast*. However, US examination demonstrates a suspicious irregular mass with heterogeneous echotexture (approximately 7 mm) at the 5 o'clock position.

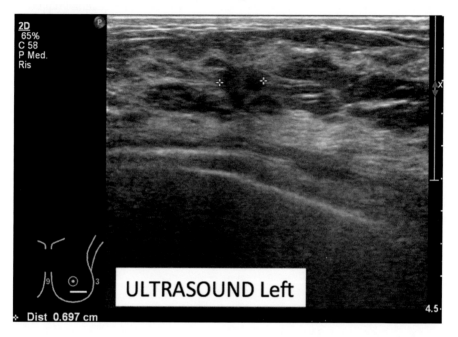

The US-guided core needle biopsy confirmed the presence of an invasive ductal carcinoma.

**MRI** No significant focal area of contrast enhancement in the right breast.

MRI confirms the presence of a cancer (10 mm) at the confluence of inner quadrants of the *left breast* (*white arrow*). A further area (*white arrow*) of contrast enhancement was detected on the same side, in the upper outer quadrant (approximately 6 mm). Biopsy confirmed a B5b lesion (invasive ductal carcinoma). No metastatic lymphadenopathy in the axillary region. (**a**) Postcontrast subtracted image. (**b**) Postcontrast maximum intensity projection image.

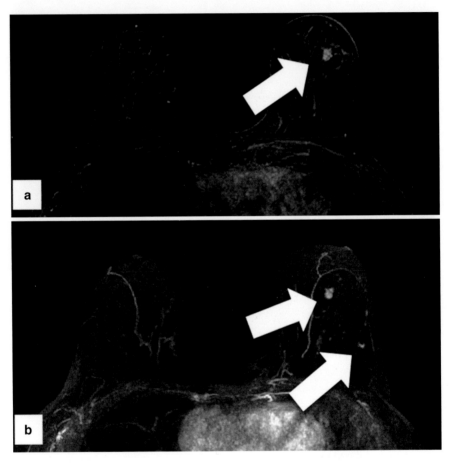

**Surgical Specimen Report** Invasive ductal carcinoma was found in the right breast.

**Conclusions** DBT allowed improved evaluation of the right architectural distortion compared to FFDM and confirmed its presence. In particular, DBT image showed an architectural distortion in the right breast not detectable on the US and MRI examination. Furthermore, US and MRI detected a mass on the left side, not detectable on DBT (on the left side) (See Video C8_RMLO).

### 5.1.9   Case 9

**Case History** Woman, 80 years old, underwent mammography for screening purposes.
   Previous surgery on the left breast.

**Mammography** Fatty breast. Right MLO FFDM image shows an architectural distortion (*white circle*) in the middle third of the superior right breast. No further suspicious findings.

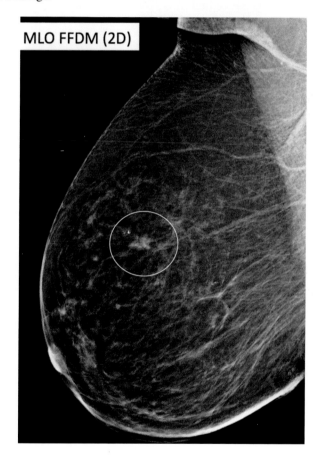

**Tomosynthesis** Right MLO DBT image confirms the presence of an architectural distortion (*white circle*), better visible on DBT than on FFDM.

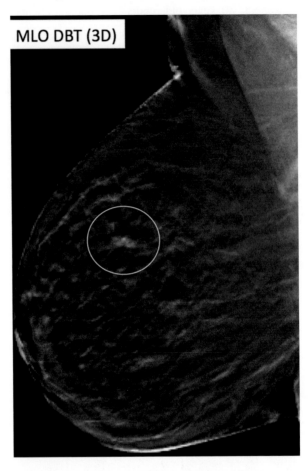

**Ultrasound** This suspicious finding is also visible at ultrasound examination. Targeted US image demonstrates a small suspicious hypoechoic mass.

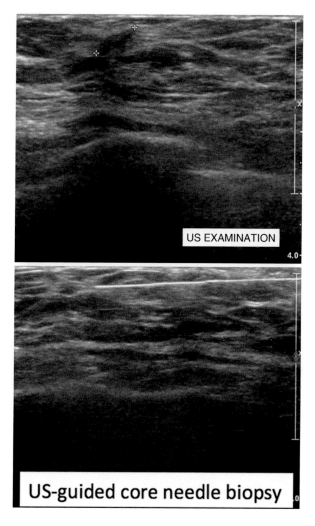

Ultrasound-guided biopsy confirmed a B5b lesion (Invasive Ductal Carcinoma).

**Conclusions** DBT allowed improved visualization of the architectural distortion (See Video C9_RMLO).

### 5.1.10 Case 10

**Case History** Woman, 72 years old, underwent mammography for screening purposes.

**Mammography** Almost entirely fatty breast. Left CC FFDM image shows a high-density irregular mass with spiculated margins (*white arrow*) in the central breast (approximately 10 mm). No further suspicious findings.

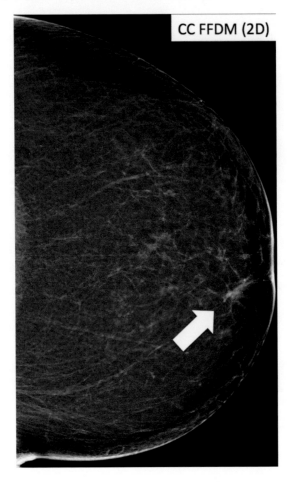

**Tomosynthesis** Left CC DBT image demonstrates the presence of an architectural distortion in the central breast (*white arrow*).

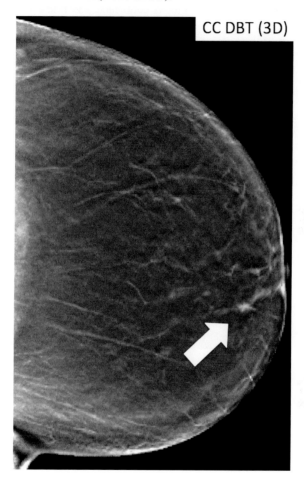

**Ultrasound** The suspicious lesion is also visible at ultrasound examination. US image shows a 5-mm hypoechoic taller-than-wide mass.

Ultrasound-guided core needle biopsy confirmed a B5b lesion (invasive ductal carcinoma).

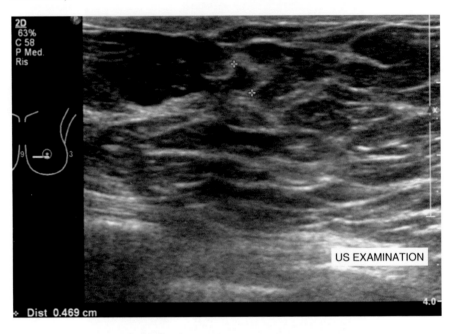

**Conclusions** DBT allowed improved evaluation of the architectural distortion.

### 5.1.11  Case 11

**Case History** Woman, 58 years old, underwent mammography for screening purposes. No symptoms. Family history was unremarkable.

**Mammography** Heterogeneously dense breast. Left CC FFDM image shows an irregular mass associated with an architectural distortion in the outer quadrants of the left breast (*white circle*).

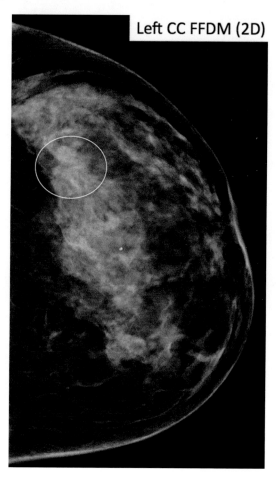

Left CC FFDM (2D)

**Tomosynthesis** DBT supports mammographic finding. The single tomosynthesis slice image of the left breast in CC view (*white circle*) shows a suspicious mass, approximately 15 mm in diameter surrounded by an architectural distortion.

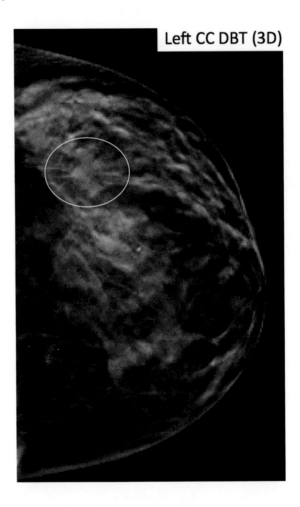

**Ultrasound**   Corresponding US image shows a mass with indistinct borders in the left breast at 3 o'clock position (13 mm diameter). US also detects a suspicious area with heterogeneous echotexture at 3 o'clock position in the *right breast* (10 mm).

The US-guided core needle biopsies confirmed an invasive ductal carcinoma in the left breast and a nonmalignant finding (fibroadenoma) in the right breast. Calipers on the US image are not measuring the lesion biopsied.

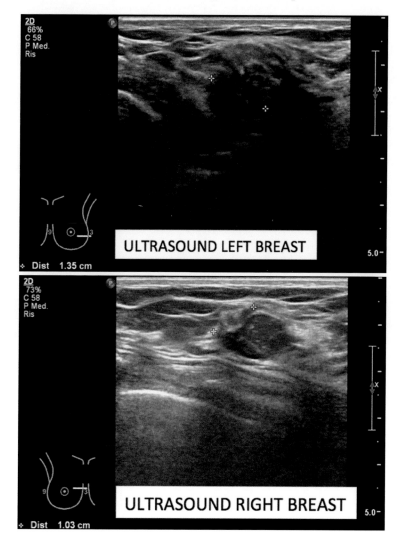

**MRI** MRI evaluation shows the mass (15 mm) in the outer quadrant of the *left* breast (*white arrow*). No further area of contrast enhancement is visible. No metastatic lymphadenopathy in the axillary region is detected.

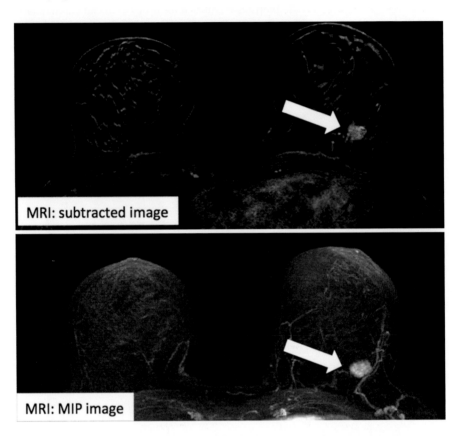

**Conclusions** DBT allowed a better evaluation of the spiculated margins of the mass on the left breast. Ultrasound gave a false positive on the right breast. In this case, on the right side, DBT avoided a biopsy of a benign lesion on the right breast (See Video C11_LCC).

### 5.1.12 Case 12

**Case History** Woman, 48 years old, underwent mammography for screening purposes. No symptoms.

**Mammography** Heterogeneously dense breast. Right MLO FFDM image shows an architectural distortion (*white circle*) in the middle third of the superior right breast.

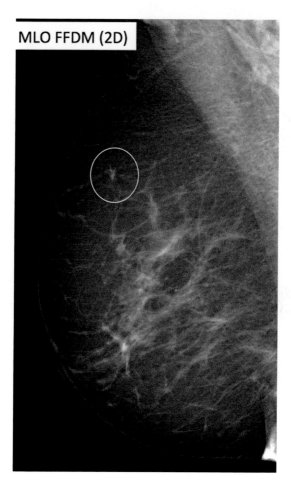

**Tomosynthesis** Right MLO DBT shows normal findings. DBT demonstrates that the pseudo-architectural distortion is caused by tissue summation (*white circle*).

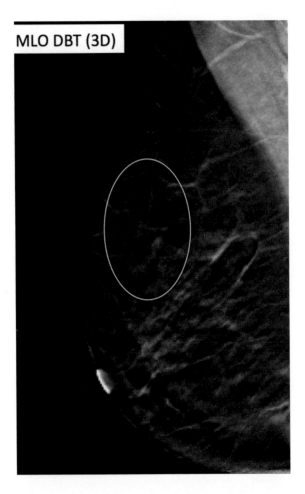

**Conclusions** DBT solved the suspicious mammographic finding and avoided further assessment.

### 5.1.13  Case 13

**Case History**  Woman, 68 years old, underwent mammography for screening purposes. Previous surgery on the left breast.

**Mammography**  Almost entirely fatty breast. Right CC FFDM image shows an architectural distortion (*white arrow*) in the lateral right breast.

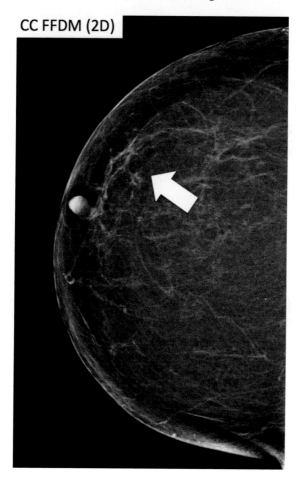

**Tomosynthesis** Single DBT image of the right breast in CC view solves the suspicious mammographic finding (*white circle*). The FFDM finding is due to tissue summation.

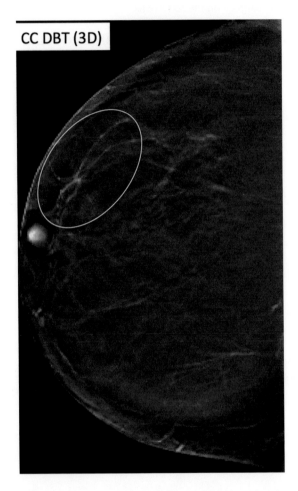

**Conclusions** DBT solved the suspicious mammographic finding and avoided further assessment. No lesions were detected at follow-up.

### 5.1.14  Case 14

**Case History**  Woman, 84 years old, who underwent mammography for spontaneous screening purposes.

**Mammography**  Heterogeneously dense breast. Right CC and MLO FFDM images show an irregular mass with associated cluster of microcalcifications (*white arrow*) in the posterior central third of the right breast.

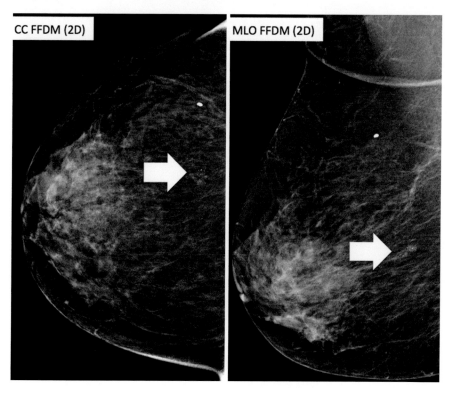

**Tomosynthesis**  Right CC and MLO DBT images support mammographic findings showing a suspicious mass with associated cluster of microcalcifications in the posterior central third of the right breast (*white arrow*). The mass margins appear more spiculated on DBT.

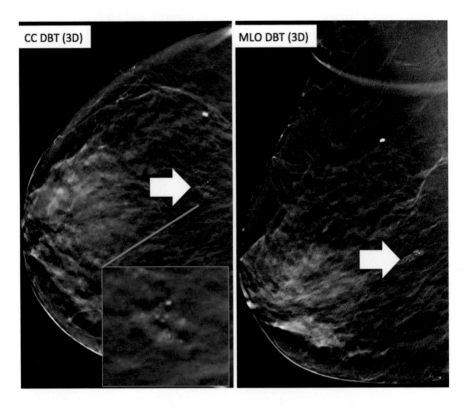

**Conclusions**  DBT confirms the presence of microcalcifications and improved visualization of the spiculated margins of the mass. See also Case 2 for microcalcification comments (See Video C14_RCC).

## Reference

Peppard HR, Nicholson BE, Rochman CM, Merchant JK, Mayo RC 3rd, Harvey JA (2015) Digital breast tomosynthesis in the diagnostic setting: indications and clinical applications. Radiographics 35(4):975–990. doi: 10.1148/rg.2015140204. Epub 2015 May 29

### 5.1.15  Case 15

**Case History**  Woman, 77 years old, underwent mammography for spontaneous screening purposes. Previous surgery on the right breast.

**Mammography**  Right CC FFDM image shows a cluster of fine microcalcifications and linear branching microcalcifications in the central breast (*white arrow*).

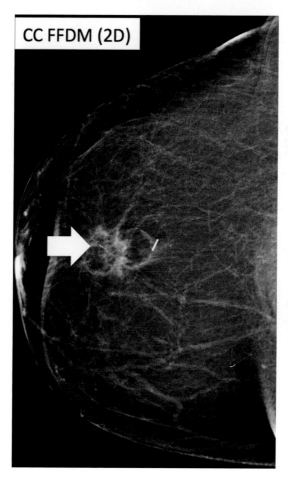

**Tomosynthesis** Right CC DBT view supports the mammographic findings and shows the cluster of microcalcifications and linear branching microcalcifications in central breast (*white arrow*).

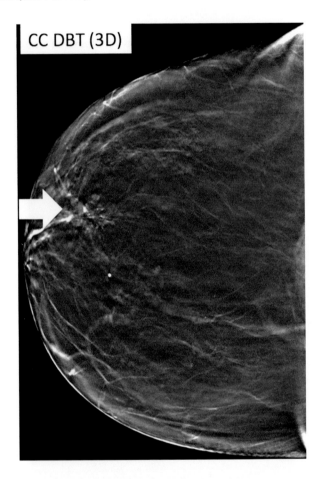

**Conclusions** DBT supports mammographic findings. IDC with in situ components was demonstrated after surgery. Liponecrosis is better shown on FFDM. On DBT, liponecrosis is difficult to be identified (See Video C15_RCC).

## 5.1.16 Case 16

**Case History** Woman, 64 years old, who underwent mammography for screening purposes.

**Mammography** Heterogeneously dense breast. Right CC FFDM image shows an architectural distortion (*white circle*) in the central breast.

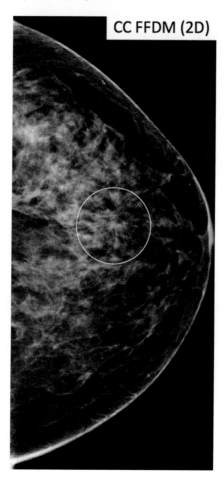

**Tomosynthesis** Right CC DBT view supports mammographic finding and shows the architectural distortion (*white circle*) in central breast.

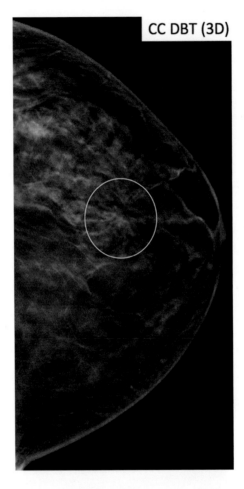

**Conclusions** DBT supports mammographic finding. DBT allows a better visualization of the architectural distortion (See Video C16_LCC).

### 5.1.17  Case 17

**Case History**  A 72-year-old woman underwent mammography for screening purposes.

**Mammography**  Right CC FFDM image shows an architectural distortion associated with cluster of microcalcifications (*white arrow*) in the outer quadrants.

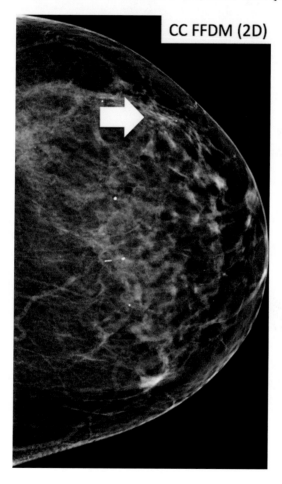

**Tomosynthesis** Right CC DBT image supports mammographic finding. DBT shows a cluster of microcalcifications (*white arrow*) in the outer quadrants and confirms the presence of the architectural distortion.

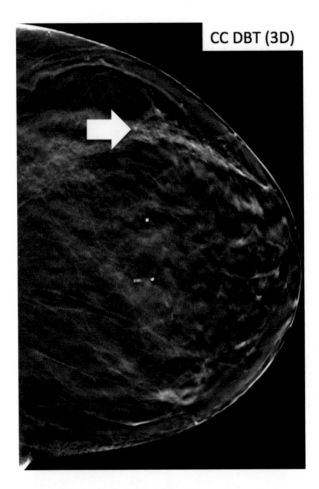

**Conclusions** DBT supports mammographic finding. An invasive ductal carcinoma was diagnosed at histologic examination (See Video C17_LCC).

### 5.1.18 Case 18

**Case History** A 64-year-old woman underwent mammography for screening purposes.

Clinical history was unremarkable.

**Mammography** Left CC and MLO FFDM image show fine microcalcifications (*white arrow*) in the posterior third of the superior right breast.

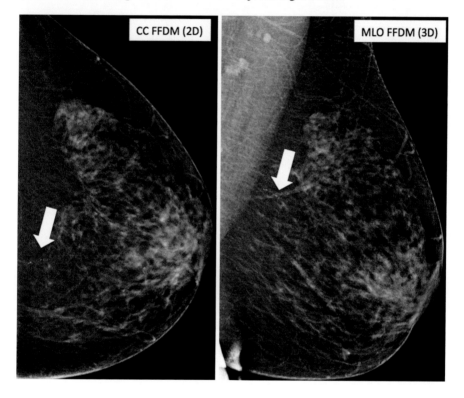

**Tomosynthesis** Left CC and MLO DBT image support mammographic finding and show cluster of microcalcifications (*white arrow*).

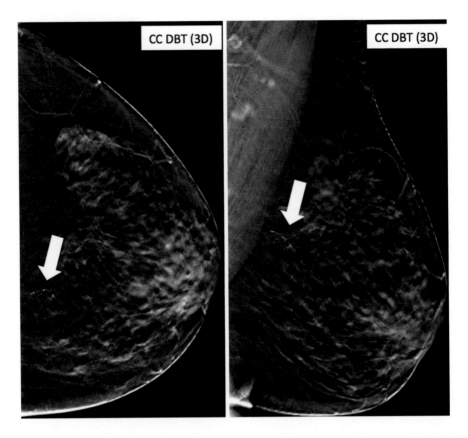

**Conclusions** DBT supports mammographic finding. The result of the histological examination was DCIS.

### 5.1.19 Case 19

**Case History** Woman, 64 years old, who underwent mammography for screening purposes.

**Mammography** Right CC FFDM image shows a suspicious low-density mass in the medial left breast (*white arrow*). No further suspicious findings are present.

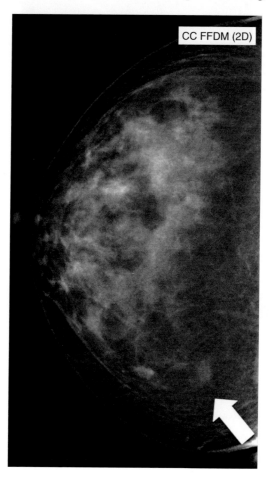

**Tomosynthesis** The suspicious mass shown on mammography is considered not visible in the inner quadrants (*white circle*). Therefore, DBT solved the suspicious mammographic finding, which was probably due to tissue summation.

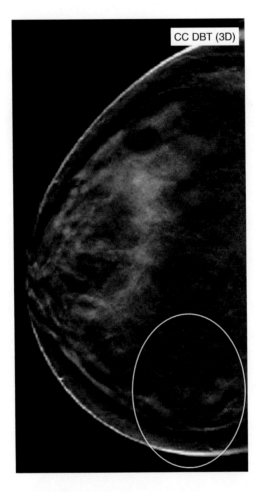

**Conclusion** In this case, DBT solved the suspicious mammographic finding avoiding a biopsy. Follow-up was negative (See Video C19c).

## 5.1.20 Case 20

**Case History** Woman, 66 years old, who underwent mammography for screening purposes.

**Mammography** Almost entirely fatty breast. Right CC FFDM shows a mass in the central breast (*white arrow*). No further suspicious findings are present.

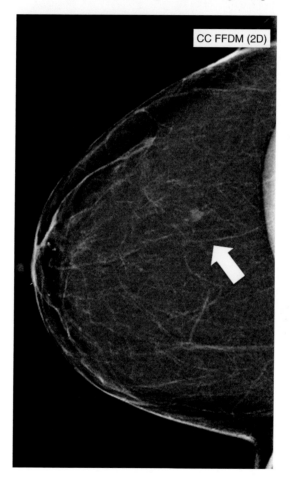

**Tomosynthesis** The nodule shown on mammography is considered not visible on DBT (*white circle*). Right MLO DBT image shows that the suspicious mammographic finding is due to tissue summation.

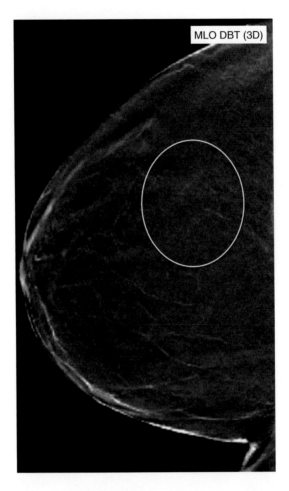

**Conclusion** In this case, DBT solved the suspicious mammographic finding avoiding a biopsy. Follow-up was negative (See Video C20c).

### 5.1.21 Case 21

**Case History** Woman, 54 years old, underwent mammography for screening purposes. No symptoms.

**Mammography** Heterogeneously dense breast. Right MLO FFDM image shows an architectural distortion in the middle third of the superior right breast (*white arrow*). No further suspicious findings are present.

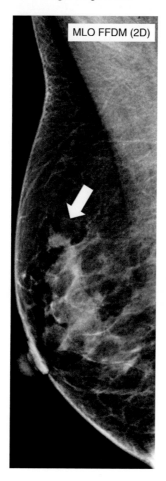

**Tomosynthesis** The suspicious finding shown on mammography is considered not visible on DBT (*white circle*). The suspicious area shown on FFDM resembles the parenchyma of the adjacent normal mammary gland. Therefore, DBT solved the suspicious mammographic finding.

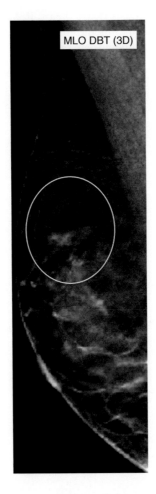

**Conclusion** In this case, DBT solved the suspicious mammographic finding avoiding a biopsy.

Follow-up was uneventful (See Video C21c).

## 5.1.22 Case 22

**Case History** Woman, 53 years old, underwent mammography for screening purposes.

**Mammography** Heterogeneously dense breast. Left MLO FFDM image shows an architectural distortion in the middle third of the superior left breast (*white arrow*). No further suspicious findings are present.

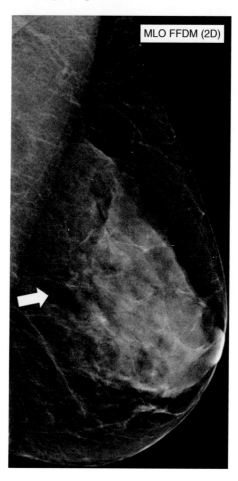

**Tomosynthesis** Left MLO DBT image shows an architectural distortion in the middle third of the left breast (*white circle*). Therefore, DBT confirmed the suspicious mammographic finding.

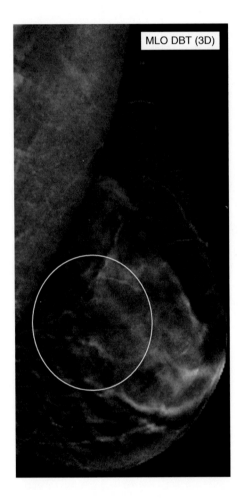

**Magnetic Resonance Imaging** MRI subtracted images don't show any area of suspicious contrast enhancement in the left breast (*white circle*).

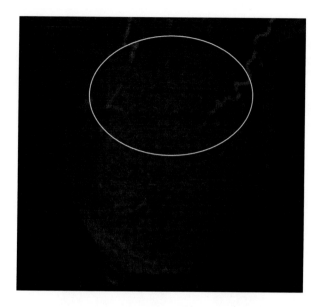

**Histological Exam** The result of surgical biopsy was usal ductal hyperplasia (UDH)

**Conclusion** In this case, DBT and FFDM show a finding not shown on MRI. However, the finding was not malignant (See Video C22_LMLO).

### 5.1.23 Case 23

**Case History** Woman, 44 years old, who underwent mammography for screening purposes.

**Mammography** Heterogeneously dense breast. Right MLO FFDM image (*white arrow*) shows a suspicious architectural distortion in the middle third of the superior right breast. No further suspicious findings are present.

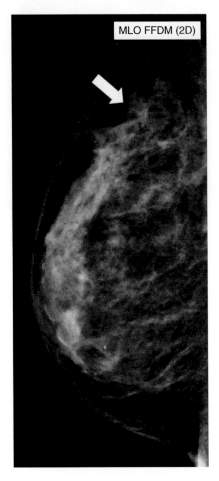

**Tomosynthesis** Right MLO DBT image confirms architectural distortion in middle
third of the superior right breast. Therefore, DBT (*white circle*) confirmed the suspicious mammographic finding.

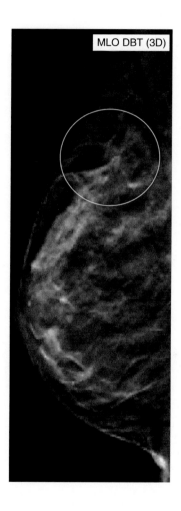

**Ultrasound** Corresponding US image confirms the presence of a small irregular hypoechoic mass in the right upper lateral quadrant (*white arrow*). In addition, US examination shows a further suspicious finding in periareolar area (*empty arrow*).

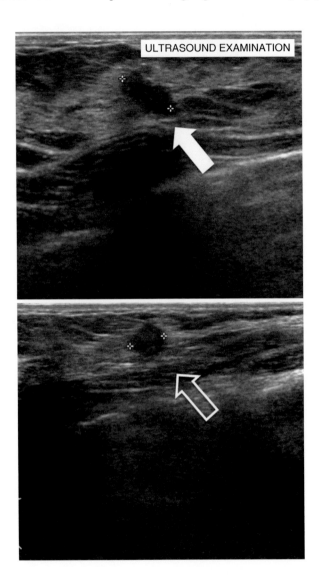

**MRI**  MRI shows two enhancing right breast masses (*white arrows*).

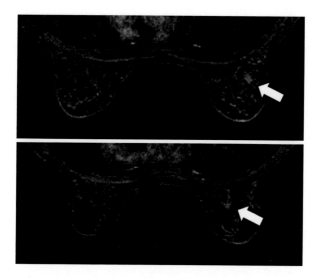

**Conclusion**  The result of the histological exam was a multicentric invasive ductal carcinoma (IDC). In this case, ultrasound and MRI showed a further finding not shown on FFDM and DBT (See Video C23_RCC).

## Reference

Yi A, Cho N, Yang KS, Han W, Noh DY, Moon WK (2015) Breast cancer recurrence in patients with newly diagnosed breast cancer without and with preoperative MR imaging: a matched cohort study. Radiology. 2015;276(3):695–705. doi: 10.1148/radiol.2015142101. Epub 2015 Apr 27.

### 5.1.24 Case 24

**Case History** Woman, 59 years old, who underwent mammography for a clinical finding. She had a mammography performed in another hospital, not conclusive, but suspicious for the presence of an architectural distortion and microcalcifications.

**Tomosynthesis** Left MLO DBT image (*white arrow*) confirms the architectural distortion associated with microcalcifications in the anterior and middle third of the superior left breast. DBT showed *only one* suspicious finding.

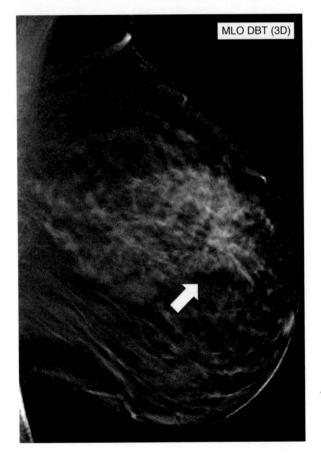

**MRI**  MRI shows two areas of contrast enhancement in the left breast (*white arrow* and *white empty arrow*).

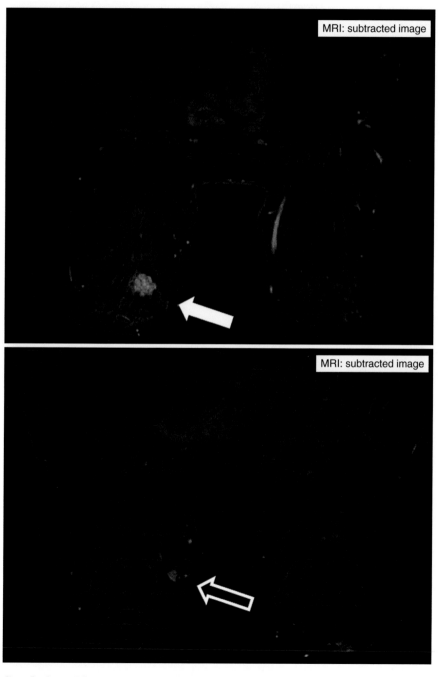

**Conclusion**  After surgery, there was a multicentric invasive ductal carcinoma (IDC). In this case, MRI showed an additional lesion not shown on DBT.

## References

Luparia A, Mariscotti G, Durando M, Ciatto S, Bosco D, Campanino PP, Castellano I, Sapino A, Gandini G (2013) Accuracy of tumor size assessment in the preoperative staging of breast cancer: comparison of digital mammography, tomosynthesis, ultrasound and MRI. Radiol Med 118(7):1119–1136. doi: 10.1007/s11547-013-0941-z. Epub 2013 Jun 25. PubMed PMID: 23801389

Mariscotti G, Houssami N, Durando M, Bergamasco L, Campanino PP, Ruggieri C, Regini E, Luparia A, Bussone R, Sapino A, Fonio P, Gandini G (2014) Accuracy of mammography, digital breast tomosynthesis, ultrasound and MR imaging in preoperative assessment of breast cancer. Anticancer Res 34(3):1219–1225. PubMed PMID: 24596363

Yi A, Cho N, Yang KS, Han W, Noh DY, Moon WK (2015) Breast cancer recurrence in patients with newly diagnosed breast cancer without and with preoperative MR imaging: a matched cohort study. Radiology 142101. [Epub ahead of print]

## 5.1.25 Case 25

**Case History** Woman, 49 years old, who underwent tomosynthesis after a suspicious but not conclusive mammography performed in another hospital.

**Tomosynthesis** CC right DBT image shows two architectural distortions (*white oval*) in the central breast beside the clip from a previous VABB (vacuum-assisted breast biopsy).

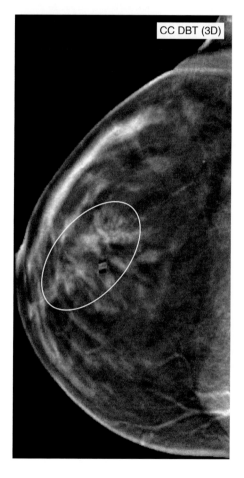

**Conclusion**  The result of histology was a radial scar. In this case, DBT shows a finding located in a critical area after a VABB, but it is not able to differentiate the radial scar from a cancer (See Video C25_RCC).

## Reference

Dominguez A, Durando M, Mariscotti G, Angelino F, Castellano I, Bergamasco L, Bianchi CC, Fonio P, Gandini G (2015) Breast cancer risk associated with the diagnosis of a microhistological radial scar (RS): retrospective analysis in 10 years of experience. Radiol Med 120(4):377–385. doi: 10.1007/s11547-014-0456-2. Epub 2014 Aug 26

### 5.1.26  Case 26

**Case History**  Woman, 58 years old, who underwent mammography for screening purposes.

**Mammography**  Heterogeneously dense breast. Right MLO FFDM image shows a mass with indistinct margins in the posterior third of the right breast (*white arrow*). No further suspicious findings are present.

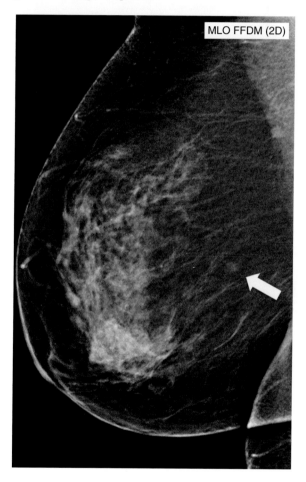

**Tomosynthesis** The nodule shown on mammography is considered not visible (*white circle*). Therefore, DBT solved the suspicious mammographic finding, which probably was due to tissue superimposition.

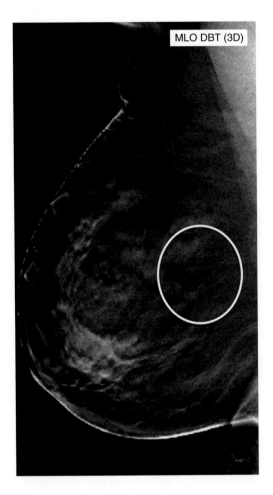

**Conclusion** In this case, DBT solved suspicious mammographic finding avoiding a biopsy. The follow-up was uneventful.

### 5.1.27  Case 27

**Case History**  Woman, 69 years old, who underwent tomosynthesis after a suspicious but not conclusive mammography performed in another hospital.

**Tomosynthesis**  Left DBT image (*white arrow*) shows a suspicious irregular mass posteriorly to a known cluster of microcalcifications in the lateral breast.

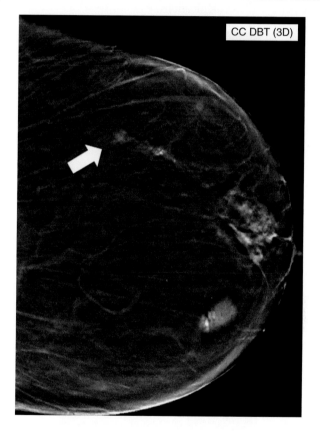

**Conclusion**  After surgery, there was an invasive ductal carcinoma (IDC). In this case, DBT shows a finding not clearly shown in the mammography as malignant.

### 5.1.28  Case 28

**Case History** Woman, 51 years old, underwent mammography for screening purposes.

**Mammography** Heterogeneously dense breast tissue. Right CC FFDM image shows an irregular mass (*white circle*) with unclear edges (8 mm) in the central breast. Diffuse benign microcalcifications.

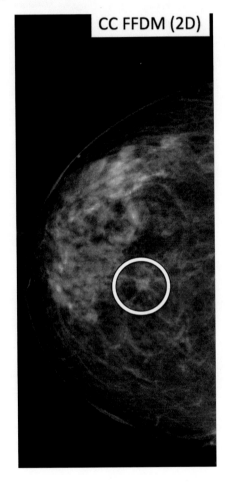

**Tomosynthesis** Right CC DBT image solved the suspicious mammographic finding (*white circle*).

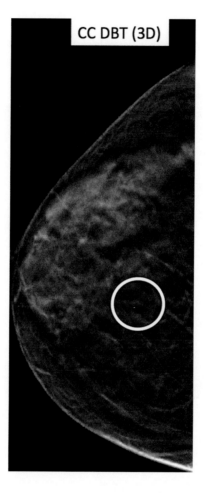

**Conclusions** The suspicious mammographic finding was caused by tissue summation. DBT solved suspicious mammographic finding (See Videos C28_RCC and C28_RMLO).

### 5.1.29 Case 29

**Case History** Woman, 55 years old, underwent mammography for screening purposes.

**Mammography** Heterogeneously dense breast tissue. Left CC FFDM image shows an architectural distortion (*white circle*) in the inner quadrants of the left breast.

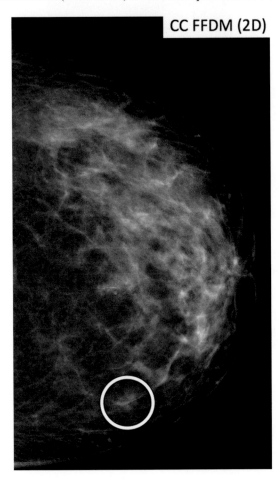

**Tomosynthesis** The suspicious architectural distortion shown on mammography in the inner quadrants is considered not visible. DBT (*white circle*) solved suspicious mammographic finding.

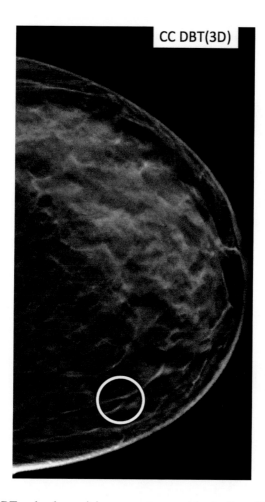

**Conclusions** DBT solved suspicious mammographic finding. The architectural distortion seen on FFDM was caused by tissue superimposition (See Video C29_LCC).

## 5.1.30 Case 30

**Case History** Woman, 65 years old, underwent mammography for screening purposes.

**Mammography** Heterogeneously dense breast tissue. Left CC FFDM image (*white circle*) shows an architectural distortion in the outer quadrants of the left breast.

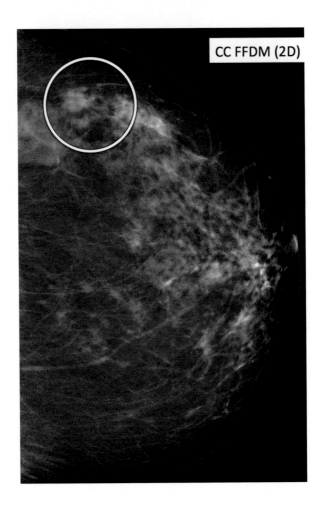

**Tomosynthesis** Left CC DBT image (*white circle*) solved the suspicious mammographic finding.

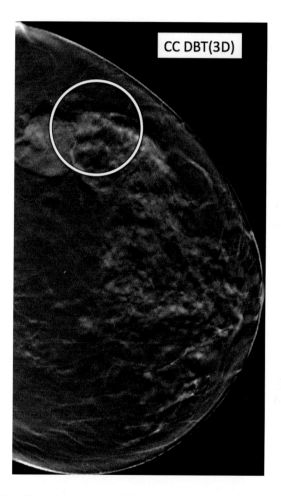

**Conclusions**  The distortion seen on FFDM was caused by tissue superimposition. DBT solved suspicious mammographic finding.

### 5.1.31 Case 31

**Case History** Woman, 47 years old, underwent mammography for screening purposes.

**Mammography** Heterogeneously dense breast tissue. Right CC FFDM image (*white circle*) shows an architectural distortion in central breast.

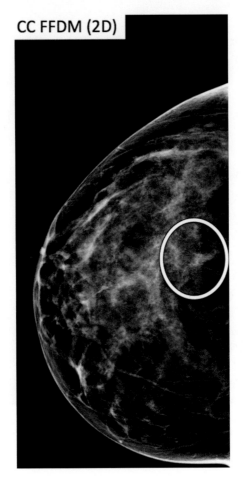

**Tomosynthesis** The suspicious architectural distortion shown (*white circle*) on mammography is considered not visible in the central breast on DBT. Therefore, DBT solved the suspicious mammographic finding.

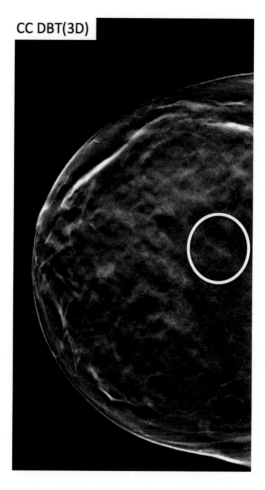

**Conclusions** In this case, DBT solved suspicious mammographic finding. The distortion seen on FFDM was caused by tissue summation (See Video C31_RCC).

### 5.1.32 Case 32

**Case History** Woman, 53 years old, underwent aimed mammography, tomosynthesis, and ultrasound examination to evaluate suspicious finding.

**Mammography** Left CC and MLO FFDM images show a suspicious architectural distortion (*white circle* and *white arrow*) in the medial and middle third of the superior left breast.

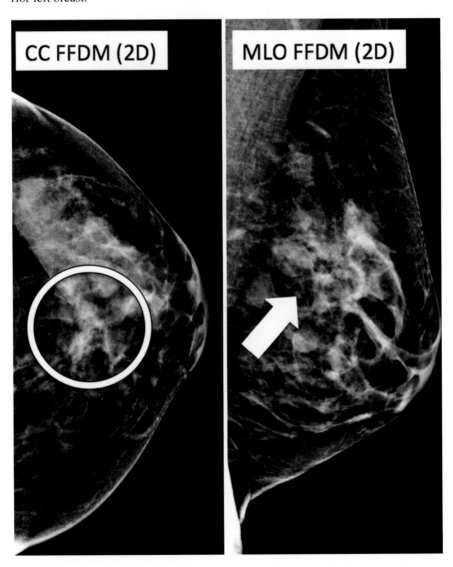

**Tomosynthesis**  Left CC and MLO DBT images confirm the suspicious architectural distortion. The suspicious finding is better visualized at DBT than at FFDM (*white circle* and *white arrow*).

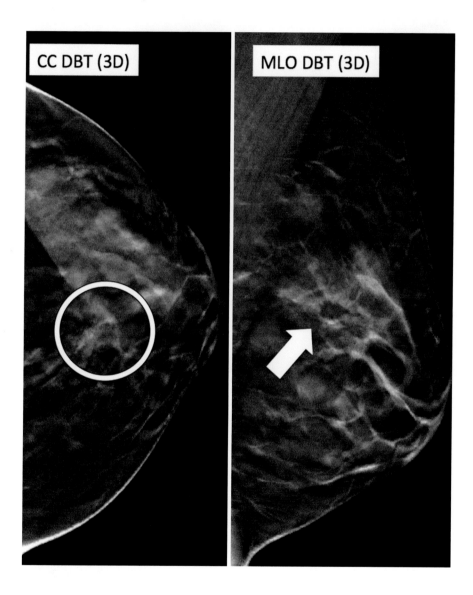

**Ultrasound**  US (*white arrow*) examination demonstrates an irregular hypoechoic mass with indistinct margins at the 11 o'clock position.

An invasive ductal carcinoma was diagnosed at histologic examination.

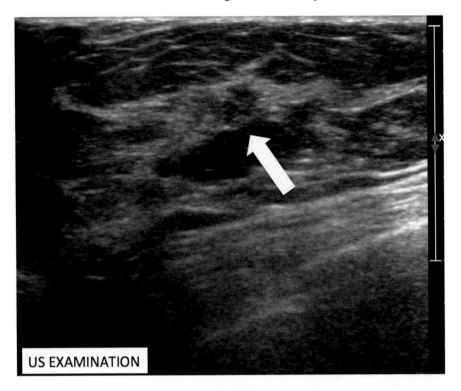

**Conclusions**  DBT allowed a better evaluation of the lesion and confirmed its presence (See Videos C32_LCC and C32_LMLO).

### 5.1.33 Case 33

**Case History** Woman, 42 years old, underwent mammography, tomosynthesis, and ultrasound examination to evaluate suspicious findings of a previous mammogram acquired in another center. A sclerosing lesion in the same breast was already known.

**Mammography and Tomosynthesis** Left CC FFDM and DBT image demonstrate two architectural distortion, the bigger one located in the outer quadrants (approximately 11 mm) and the other one, smaller (approximately 9 mm), in inner quadrants(*white circles*).

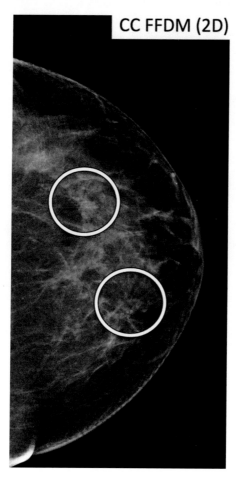

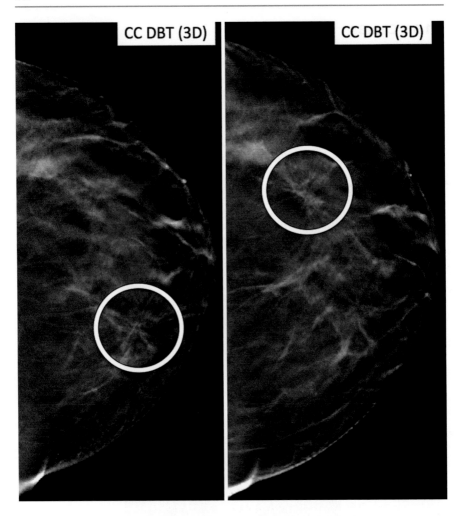

The first one is also visible at ultrasound examination and has already been biopsied (sclerosing lesion); the latter one is not visible at ultrasound examination.

Stereotactic VABB of the architectural distortion at inner quadrants gave the following histological result: B3 lesion – papillary lesion with sclerosing adenosis.

**Conclusions** FFDM and DBT allowed detection of a lesion not visible at US.

### 5.1.34  Case 34

**Case History** Woman, 45 years old, underwent mammography for screening purposes.

**Mammography** Scattered fibroglandular tissue. Left CC FFDM image shows a focal asymmetry (*white arrow*) in the central breast.

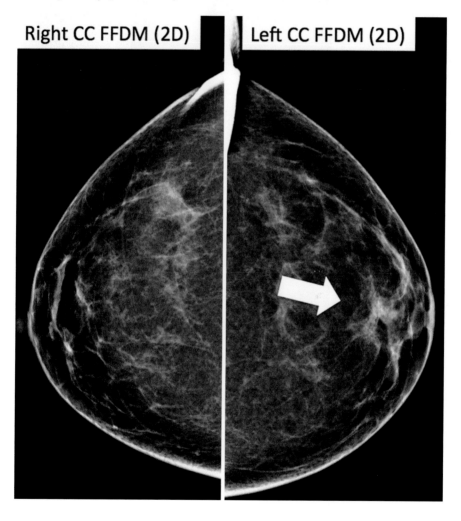

Right CC FFDM (2D)    Left CC FFDM (2D)

**Tomosynthesis** Left CC DBT image (*white oval*) shows normal findings. The suspicious finding shown on FFDM is considered not visible in the central breast. Therefore, DBT solved the suspicious mammographic finding.

Follow-up was negative.

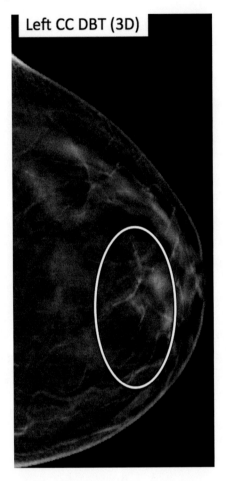

**Conclusions** DBT solved suspicious mammographic finding caused by tissue summation (See Video C34_LCC).

### 5.1.35  Case 35

**Case History** Woman, 46 years old, underwent mammography for screening purposes.

**Mammography** Heterogeneously dense breast tissue. Left MLO FFDM image shows a mass/architectural distortion (*white circle*) in the middle third of the left breast.

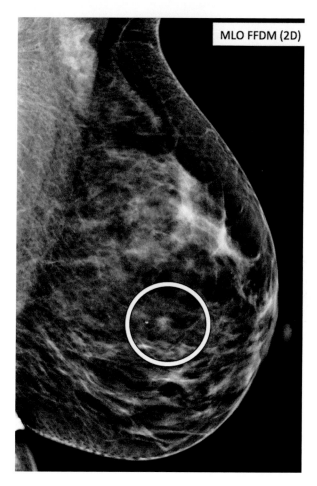

**Tomosynthesis**   Left MLO DBT image solved suspicious mammographic findings (*white circle*). The mammographic findings are due to tissue superimposition.

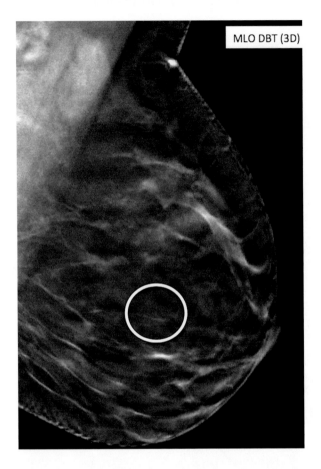

**Conclusions**   DBT solved suspicious mammographic findings.

## 5.1.36  Case 36

**Case History** Woman, 42 years old, underwent mammography for screening purposes.

**Mammography** Scattered areas of fibroglandular dense breast. Left CC FFDM image shows a focal asymmetry (*white arrow*) in outer quadrants.

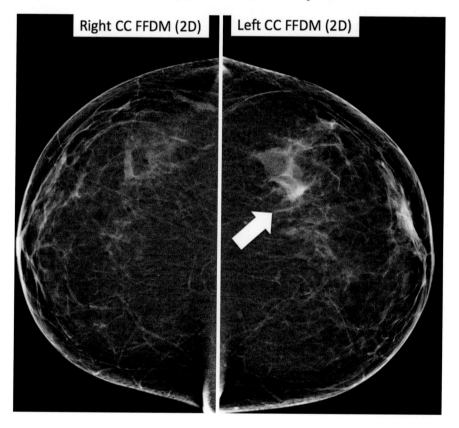

**Tomosynthesis** Left CC DBT image shows normal findings.

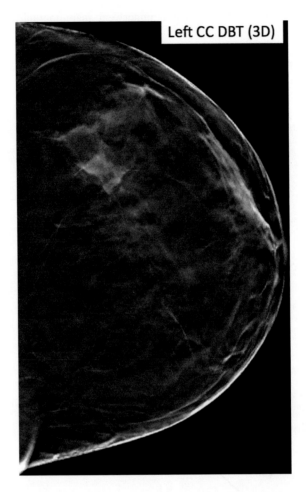

Left CC DBT (3D)

**Conclusions** DBT reclassify the mammographic finding as benign finding (normal breast tissue) (See Video C36_LCC).

### 5.1.37 Case 37

**Case History** Woman, 50 years old, underwent mammography for screening purposes.

**Mammography** Heterogeneously dense breast. CC FFDM image shows an irregular mass (approximately 12 mm) in the medial breast (*white arrow*).

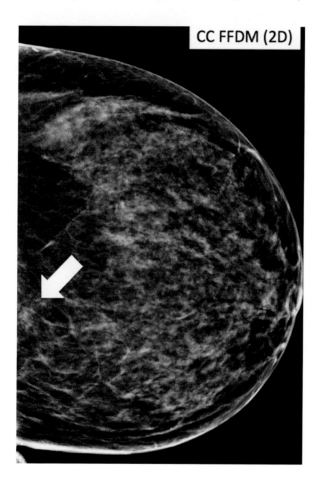

**Tomosynthesis** CC DBT image solved suspicious mammographic finding (*white arrow*).

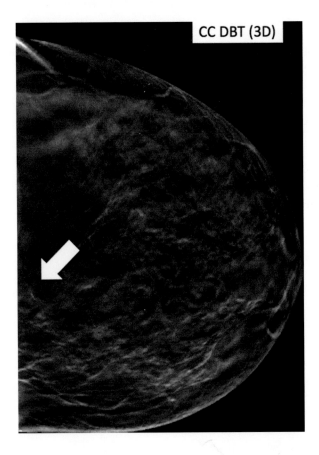

**Conclusions** DBT solved suspicious mammographic finding due to tissue superimposition.